EARLY PRAISE FOR *EARLY DETECTION*

"I've spent the last twenty-five years trying to convey exactly what this deeply personal, insightful and well reported book shouts, that detecting cancers early, when they are the most treatable, is the key to saving countless lives. It is what policymakers need to hear."

—**KATIE COURIC**
AWARD-WINNING JOURNALIST, *NEW YORK TIMES* BEST-SELLING AUTHOR
OF *GOING THERE* AND CO-FOUNDER OF STAND UP TO CANCER

"This powerful book makes a decisive argument that our current strategy against cancer would be vastly enhanced if tumors were detected at earlier stages. I wish that every patient, and policy maker, would read and understand the broad implications of this invaluable, highly readable book."

—**SIDDHARTHA MUKHERJEE, MD**
CANCER RESEARCHER AND PULITZER PRIZE-WINNING AUTHOR OF
THE EMPEROR OF ALL MALADIES: A BIOGRAPHY OF CANCER

"My mother died from breast cancer when I was 11 and there is not a day that I don't wish we had detected it sooner. This book is an engaging, informative and hugely important work that will save lives, especially if policy makers take up the authors' plea to fund more early detection testing."

—**KEN BURNS**
GRAMMY AND EMMY AWARD-WINNING
DOCUMENTARY FILMMAKER

"*Early Detection* provides an important look into testing and treatment disparities that exist in cancer care, and thoughtful guidance about how to mitigate these inequities. Expanding access is in everyone's best interest as it has the potential to increase the chance of survival while lowering the cost of care."

—**SELWYN M. VICKERS, MD**
PRESIDENT AND CEO,
MEMORIAL SLOAN-KETTERING CANCER CENTER

"This powerful book gives us real hope that we can slash tragically high cancer death rates by expanding early detection testing, and especially by ending the terrible disparities in screening and treatment rates. This is a manifesto for a positive new era in cancer care."

—JESSICA M. BIBLIOWICZ
CHAIRMAN OF THE BOARD OF FELLOWS, WEILL CORNELL MEDICINE

"In clear and compelling arguments, this book proposes an exciting, three-part plan for increasing the scope and accuracy of cancer screening, which could safely reduce cancer death rates by as much as two-thirds if widely-available, free, and targeted to high-risk populations."

—PETER T. SCARDINO, MD
FORMER CHAIRMAN, DEPARTMENT OF SURGERY,
MEMORIAL SLOAN-KETTERING CANCER CENTER

"This terrific book is a real tour de force, It is so right that we could have a huge impact on people's health and longevity if everyone utilized cancer screening tools and if we commit to the research to develop better tools to detect more cancers in their early stages."

—LISA M. DEANGELIS, MD
CHIEF PHYSICIAN EXECUTIVE AND SCOTT M. AND LISA G. STUART CHAIR
MEMORIAL SLOAN-KETTERING CANCER CENTER

"This book is a very well-crafted tour de force. With depth and insight, the authors offer a powerful argument for how we can save thousands of lives every year with early detection screening."

—LAWRENCE SCHWARTZ, MD
CHAIRMAN OF THE DEPARTMENT OF RADIOLOGY,
MEMORIAL SLOAN-KETTERING CANCER CENTER

"This inspirational book provides compelling evidence not just for the need to prioritize early detection but to address the widening gap in healthcare disparities suffered by under-resourced communities."

—AUGUSTINE M.K. CHOI, MD
STEPHEN AND SUZANNE WEISS DEAN, WEILL CORNELL MEDICINE,
AND PROVOST FOR MEDICAL AFFAIRS, CORNELL UNIVERSITY (2017-2022)

"The passion and enlightening prose in this book illuminate this complex topic in an understandable, gripping fashion, especially the need to eliminate the disparities in who gets the best screening and treatment. It's time to change the paradigm of cancer treatment to prioritize early detection, when the battle can be won."

—PHILIP STIEG, MD
CHAIRMAN OF THE DEPARTMENT OF NEUROLOGICAL SURGERY,
WEILL CORNELL MEDICINE AND NEUROSURGEON-IN-CHIEF,
NEW YORK-PRESBYTERIAN/WEILL CORNELL MEDICAL CENTER

"This book is hopefully the catalyst for more rapid adoption of essential early detection tests, especially for lung cancer, where I have seen too many die needlessly. This will bring awareness of the need for moving quickly to embrace life-saving screening innovations."

—CLAUDIA I. HENSCHKE, PHD, MD
PROFESSOR OF DIAGNOSTIC, INTERVENTIONAL, AND MOLECULAR
RADIOLOGY, ICAHN SCHOOL OF MEDICINE AT MOUNT SINAI

"This scientifically rich book powerfully articulates what we have long known, that early detection is the best chance at curing cancer. And by addressing disparities in access to screening, even more lives will be saved in underserved and disadvantaged communities. We must heed this call to action."

—ROBERT J. MIN, MD, MBA
PRESIDENT AND CEO, WEILL CORNELL MEDICINE PHYSICIANS
ORGANIZATION AND CHAIR, DEPARTMENT OF RADIOLOGY

"This is a masterful book, which covers the political, financial, and societal issues surrounding cancer screening so astutely. It is a must-read for all investigators working on early cancer detection and prevention."

—STEVEN H. ITZKOWITZ, MD
PROFESSOR OF MEDICINE, ONCOLOGICAL SCIENCES
& MEDICAL EDUCATION AT ICAHN SCHOOL OF MEDICINE AT MOUNT SINAI,
AND CHAIR, AMERICAN CANCER SOCIETY
NATIONAL COLORECTAL CANCER ROUNDTABLE

"*Early Detection* moves briskly from cancer screening to a blueprint for improving and expanding testing. Though grounded in decades worth of useful cancer statistics, the book is readable, succinct and, most importantly, focused on the patient."

—KENT SEPKOWITZ, MD
DEPUTY PHYSICIAN-IN-CHIEF, QUALITY & SAFETY,
MEMORIAL SLOAN-KETTERING CANCER CENTER

"This book lays out both the challenges and opportunities around early detection for cancer. Readable yet rigorous, it tells a compelling story of how we have failed and where we can do better in future for all the patients we serve."

—GERALDINE McGINTY, MD, MBA, FACR
E. DARRACOTT VAUGHAN, JR., M.D. SENIOR ASSOCIATE DEAN FOR
CLINICAL AFFAIRS, PROFESSOR OF CLINICAL RADIOLOGY AND
POPULATION HEALTH SCIENCES, WEILL CORNELL MEDICINE

"Drawing on success stories with cervical, lung, prostate, and colon cancer, [Ratner and Bonislawski] provide clear examples of effective screening programs that have reduced not only overall cancer mortality but also healthcare disparities. A wonderful voice of optimism, balanced caution, and a path forward."

—JOSÉ GASTON GUILLEM, MD
CHIEF, DIVISION OF GASTROINTESTINAL SURGERY,
ROSCOE BENNETT GRAY COWPER, MD,
DISTINGUISHED PROFESSOR, UNC SCHOOL OF MEDICINE

A highly insightful and engaging book that uncovers a relatively ignored strategy in our fight against cancer – early detection. The suggestions on policy change and the barriers to overcome should be a must read for patients, providers, and policy makers."

—BRADLEY B. PUA, MD
DIRECTOR OF THE LUNG CANCER SCREENING PROGRAM,
- CHIEF, DIVISION OF INTERVENTIONAL RADIOLOGY,
- DIRECTOR, RADIOLOGY CONSULTATION SERVICES
WEILL CORNELL MEDICINE

EARLY
DETECTION

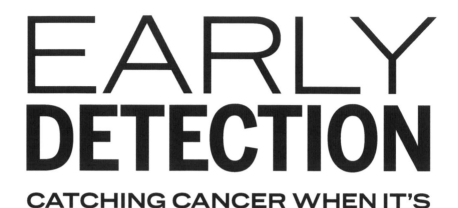

EARLY DETECTION

CATCHING CANCER WHEN IT'S CURABLE

BRUCE RATNER AND **ADAM BONISLAWSKI**

O/R

OR Books
New York · London

Published by OR Books, New York and London

Visit our website at www.orbooks.com

All rights information: rights@orbooks.com

First printing 2024

Cataloging-in-Publication data is available from the
Library of Congress.

A catalog record for this book is available from the British Library.

Cover illustration by
Frank Gehry

Cover and interior designed by
Bonnie Siegler, 8point5.com

hardback ISBN 978-1-68219-351-8
ebook ISBN 978-1-68219-352-5

Dedicated to the memory of Michael Ratner

CONTENTS

WE KNOW HOW TO STOP MANY CANCERS, SO WHY AREN'T WE?

WHEN MY BROTHER BROKE THE NEWS OF HIS DIAGNOSIS, I FELT my world falling apart. It was August 2015, and I was in Los Angeles on business. The initial call I received from my brother, Michael, was only modestly worrying. We had been exceptionally close in childhood and even more as adults. He was eighteen months older and exemplified what to me was a model of how life ought to be lived, with a moral compass that always pointed true north. He was a brilliant lawyer who had dedicated his career and remarkable capabilities to social justice and helping the oppressed. He was a principled radical, proudly so, and tireless in the human rights battles he waged. We laughed like kids when we were together and I, ever the starry-eyed younger brother, was inspired by his passion in pursuing the causes that defined his life. We shared everything.

Michael had first reached me to say he had been suddenly ill and thought it might be food poisoning. I was a board member at Weill Cornell Medicine, the superb medical school in New York City, and referred him to an infectious disease specialist there. I thought little of it until the early hours of the following morning when Michael called again to say that he had been seized by nausea so extreme he had rushed to the emergency room. Searching for the root of his illness, he said, the doctors had conducted a CT scan. Then the news. They found a brain tumor.

Like many who find themselves suddenly struggling to support a family member with a cancer diagnosis, I tried to push my emotions aside and threw myself into reading what I could on his disease, grasping at every positive sign. The tumor, Michael had said, was on his medulla, an enormously sensitive area at the base of the brain that controls essential body functions like heartbeat, breathing, and blood pressure—and yet, the doctor believed it was operable. I read that some of these tumors were troublesome but did not kill. Surely that would be the case with Michael.

I held on to my hopes, but the painful news came in waves of shock and grief. Michael was soon taken in for surgery; afterward, the doctor told us he had successfully removed the tumor spotted in the CT scan, and also found a second that could not be removed. There was more, however. The doctor determined they were metastatic malignancies from a primary tumor somewhere else in Michael's body that they were unable to locate. It was not only spreading, but, we were told, in its march through Michael's body the cancer had also gotten into his spinal fluid, and was coating his brain in a crystalline sheath. I read up on the condition, called leptomeningeal disease, and was devastated to learn that it generally leads to death within a few months.

I also sat on the board of the Memorial Sloan-Kettering Cancer Center in New York City, and so I sought out the exceptionally talented physician in chief at the time, José Baselga, to seek help with Michael's treatment. Baselga had already been engaged in a pioneering project of sequencing the genes of the tumors found at the cancer center so that they would no longer be categorized just by the organs in which they originated—an imprecise approach used for decades that, we now know, often led to fruitless treatments. Instead, they would be categorized by the specific genetic mutations that led to their uncontrolled growth and vicious attacks on their hosts. That new method opened the door, at least in theory, to far more precise targeting of the malignant cancer cells, a scalpel approach rather than the sledgehammer treatments used in many instances.

Baselga's team sequenced the genetic makeup of the cells found in Michael's tumor and discovered two prominent mutations—typically, there are dozens of mutations, if not more, in cancer patients—for which there were already government-approved therapies. Quickly, he prescribed cabozantinib, targeting what is known as the RET mutation, and Herceptin, targeting the HER2 mutation. The response was remarkable. Within days, Michael was able to stay awake for longer periods of time. We could carry on conversations as he pulled himself up in his hospital bed to greet visitors. Our hopes rose.

Soon, Michael's strength returned. He could stand and he even took an occasional assisted stroll through the corridors. We were delighted and stunned when we were told that Michael could head home just two weeks after starting the treatments. We felt we were experiencing a miracle, a tribute to the genius of modern medicine and innovations in the treatment of advanced cancers.

But we soon learned why cancer is perhaps one of the cruelest of diseases, if not the cruelest. We spent happy months together as Michael continued a variety of treatments, including chemotherapy, which was very harsh but apparently lifesaving. He devoted time to his family and was able to work on a memoir describing his achievements fighting injustice around the world. But one day Michael passed out and we rushed him to the hospital. The doctors found a dangerous infection. His body, badly weakened by the cancer and the medications keeping it at bay, was unable to overcome the spreading infection. The doctors tried to treat it, but it overwhelmed him. He died on May 11, 2016, eight months after his initial diagnosis. He was 72.

For me, the loss was profoundly painful and humbling. My position gave us access to the most thoughtful and thorough care possible, but all that had done was win us a few more months with Michael, time that was enormously precious but also frustrating. I was racked by questions about why the medical profession had not advanced further in developing cures for this terrible disease. The questions were even more piercing because this was not my family's first encounter with cancer, nor the first time our hopes had been raised only to be destroyed by a losing battle. Too many times I have felt lost due to the cruelty of cancer, then recovered and found my bearings only to have it happen again.

The experiences started when I was just 5 years old, in 1950, when my mother told Michael and me that we were going to have to share a bedroom for a while, as we had when we were younger, because our grandmother was ill and needed to stay with us. She explained that all of us were going to have to chip in and help take care of my grandmother. A hospital bed was brought in and a record player was set up next to it so we could play my grandmother's favorite song, "It's Magic," a hit from the 1940s by Doris Day. I would sit by the side of her bed and talk to her but, deeply ill by this time, all she could usually do was mumble a few incoherent words in response.

I learned only later that she had stomach cancer and had come to our home to live out her few remaining days. She died toward the end of

August, and I experienced for the first time the Jewish funeral traditions of covering all the mirrors in the house as we sat shiva, the practice of receiving family and friends for seven days of mourning. Sadly, there would be more funerals.

My father, who had lived with poor health for years, died of a heart attack when I was still a teenager. The darkness of death came to my family again in the summer of 1973, when I was 28 years old. My mother had remarried and I received a call one day from my stepfather saying that my mother had been taken in for emergency surgery for a digestive system issue. I rushed to the hospital and waited anxiously with my stepfather for news. After a few hours, the surgeon came out and told us that my mother had a complete intestinal blockage. The cause, he explained, was cancer. That frightening word again. But he said he had been able to cut out the cancerous section and that my mother had a good prognosis. We felt optimistic.

My mother came home a week later. Then began a depressing medical odyssey that many families experience. Feeling anxious and eager to understand her disease and prospects better, I went to the Cornell Medical School library and started researching invasive colon cancer. I was shocked by what I found. Despite the doctor's positive comments, I discovered that the five-year survival rate for the disease in that advanced state was less than 15 percent. The blunt truth, I realized, was that my mother was unlikely to live much longer. Knowing how hard this would hit my family, I kept the information to myself.

Over the next few years, my mother experienced additional blockages and abdominal pain. She was in and out of the hospital for more surgeries. The doctor told us these symptoms were caused by "adhesions," scar tissue that often follows abdominal surgery. I knew that was possible, but I understood that more than likely this signaled new cancerous growths. My mother endured many debilitating bouts of chemotherapy that just added to her torment with alternating periods of mental agitation and, due to the harsh treatments, breaks in her brittle bones. She died three years after her diagnosis. She was 56 years old.

Still, cancer was not through with us. In 1989, thirteen years after losing my mother, my sister-in-law Ellen, who was 36 years old and had just had her first child, a daughter, was diagnosed with breast cancer.

Though it was already a stage III cancer, her doctor, the renowned Memorial Sloan-Kettering oncologist Larry Norton, was initially optimistic.

Dr. Norton recommended the use of high-dose chemotherapy/hematopoietic stem cell transplantation (HDT/HCT). In this treatment, doctors take and store stem cells from a patient's bone marrow. Then, the patient is subjected to unusually intense chemotherapy treatments. The idea is that the patient, given doses of chemo medications normally too toxic for the body to endure, can recover afterward when the harvested healthy stem cells are reintroduced. The hope is that this sequence will kill more of the cancer cells. The side effects, however, are often horrendous: vomiting, diarrhea, exhaustion, and pain. We felt it was worth a try, though there was only limited evidence supporting the effectiveness of this treatment. In fact, that protocol has been largely abandoned today as a breast cancer treatment.

Our hopes were dashed as the disease continued its ruthless attack on Ellen. The cancer traveled to her hip, causing a broken bone and requiring a hip replacement. She had multiple hospital admissions for additional surgeries and treatment of side effects. In January 1995, despite Ellen's illness, we took a family vacation to Florida with the consent of her doctors. But once we got there, she developed a severe cough and had difficulty breathing. We rushed to an emergency room, where we received the crushing news that the cancer had metastasized and was in her lungs. We were in shock.

When we were able to bring her home, my brother-in-law, Hugo, met with Dr. Norton and was informed that Ellen had only a few months to live. She died on April 11, 1994, at 42, leaving behind a 6-year-old daughter. She was beloved and had battled heroically through the immense pain, but the best that medicine had to offer came up woefully short.

I write of my family history not because it is unique, but because it is not. This has been our shared destiny in the modern era. For men, there is roughly a one-in-two chance that they will develop cancer in their lifetime and a one-in-three chance for women, according to the NCI. We hope that we are not stricken with this terrible disease, or that loved ones are spared, but we often feel defenseless before cancer's relentless pursuit. We wrote this book to advocate for an approach that does not rely on hope as a principal defense. There is a better way.

The answer is early detection.

When I look back and recall the anguish of my many experiences with cancer—no different from that of many Americans today—it is clear to me that at least two of my family members, and perhaps more, might have been spared those tormented experiences if they had had access to what are today widely available but tragically underappreciated and underutilized areas of cancer care: screening tests that allow for early detection.

Early detection, a critical solution to the cancer epidemic, is hiding in plain sight. We have many excellent tests for screening early-stage cancers that, for a variety of reasons, have either been neglected, implemented in a haphazard way, or badly underfunded. There are some success stories that have, unquestionably, saved tens of thousands of people from dying early deaths, but too few. It is a medical system failure that this book hopes to help correct by arguing for a major expansion of early-detection programs.

In addition, as we will explain, researchers have been developing a new generation of blood-based early-detection tests that offer the hope that a single draw of blood could allow doctors to test for dozens of different cancers, most of which now elude us in their earliest stages, when they are far easier to treat and cure. Together, more intensive application of these screening technologies—and guaranteeing essential follow-up treatment for patients—represent a necessary revolution, requiring new policies and priorities. Emphasizing early detection and guaranteed treatment will provide a healthy dose of optimism that has been missing from many of our battles with cancer.

We have devoted several years to researching the issue, the challenges of the past and the promising new technologies of the future, and interviewed more than a hundred talented doctors, researchers and administrators who are involved in the field, all in the hope that we can both provide new encouragement in the war on cancer and persuade policymakers to make early detection a much greater priority.

The benefits are clear. In 1994, the year before my sister-in-law died, the BRCA1 gene and its link to breast cancer was discovered. Mutations in that gene, we learned, can be passed down through families, giving women up to an 85 percent lifetime risk of developing breast cancer.

After Ellen's death, we had her BRCA1 gene sequenced from tissue that had been preserved and found that she, indeed, was positive for a pathogenic mutation. Further, we discovered that her paternal grandmother had died at a young age from breast cancer, as had a paternal aunt.

Today, with that family history, Ellen would probably be screened for the BRCA1 mutations and, finding their presence, she likely would have had more frequent mammograms to detect tumors or would have undergone a preventive mastectomy. It might have saved her life.

Similarly, had colorectal cancer screening been commonplace fifty years ago, my mother's tumor might have been detected while it was still in a precancerous state. Today, that is common. Her doctor would have been able to remove it and it would never have bothered her again. The five-year survival rate for late-stage colorectal cancer is low and has barely budged since my mother was diagnosed, but the overall death rate from the disease has been cut almost in half because of the early screening and removal of those early-stage lesions.

All these painful experiences contributed to the sobering journey I pledged to take after my brother's death in which I confronted, with sadness but deep determination, the truth that the medical profession has failed in its battles to "cure" cancer or bring us closer to a statistical victory in our "war on cancer." I owe it to my brother and other lost family members, as well as the millions who have one of the many related diseases we group together as cancer, to understand how we might do better—not in ten or twenty years, but now.

BATTLING A "WAR" ON THE WRONG FRONT

The "war on cancer" was started by President Nixon a half-century ago; we have spent hundreds of billions of dollars on research, some of it conducted by the greatest scientific minds of our time, the recipients of many Nobel prizes for their breakthroughs; and yet, a careful analysis of the numbers makes clear that we have barely moved the needle in reducing deaths from advanced metastatic cancers through improved treatments.

Where there has been progress in treating advanced cancers, it has often "succeeded" by adding just a few months to the lives of those with the disease, as was the case with my brother. And many of those months are spent in anguish as the harsh treatments and the cancers ravage the bodies and defenses of the patients. Those are not cures.

I have read studies and books, consulted with experts and reflected. I have enormous respect for the hard work and the capabilities of the doctors who throw themselves into this effort. But I have come to the conclusion that our priorities in researching and treating cancer are badly misguided and, sadly, lead to tens of thousands of needless early deaths a year.

I am writing this book because it is time for policymakers to confront this stark truth and embrace early detection with a spirit of energy and innovation. We need to flip our decades-long priority of focusing largely on the treatment of advanced cancers—often in stage III or stage IV—and shift the emphasis to early detection of cancerous growths, until now the poor stepchild of the whole process. While it will remain vital that we continue to study and aggressively treat advanced cancers to the best of our abilities, the underfunded early-detection technologies and provisions for necessary treatment of the malignancies they find will save far more lives more quickly, particularly for lower-income patients.

This book explains that our challenge as a society isn't just confronting the extreme, pernicious nature of cancer, but the simple fact that we've been looking for solutions in the wrong place. I am urging not an either/or switch, but a rebalancing of the focus of our healthcare priorities, our public healthcare policies, and where we apply our billions of research dollars.

We must launch a campaign to bring early-detection screening to more people, particularly lower-income people and people of color who are too often overlooked in our healthcare system, and to developing new early-detection tests that could transform our ability to defeat cancers before they spread. The payoff, in the form of lives saved, potential reductions in healthcare costs, increased economic activity, and families kept intact, would be immense.

Adding to the growing need to do a better job of preventing and curing cancers is the stark reality that the U.S. population is aging, and fast. This is important because the probability of getting cancer rises rapidly with age. The older we get, the more vulnerable we become to developing various cancers and the harder it gets to stop them.

According to Census Bureau figures, the number of people in the U.S. age 65 and older will rise to 96 million by 2060 from 52 million in 2018. That will trigger a spike in cancer given that, for those under the age of 20, the incidence of cancer is fewer than 25 cases per 100,000 population, which rises to 350 cases for the 45–49 age range and 1,000 cases for those 60 and older, according to NCI data. As a result, the Centers for Disease Control and Prevention forecasts that the incidence of cancer in the U.S. will jump to 2.3 million in 2050 from 1.5 million in 2015. Adding to the challenge is the fact, since around 1990, more young people have been developing cancers, perhaps due to changes in diet, lifestyle, the environment and obesity rates.

Applying the early-detection technologies we already have in more comprehensive ways—everything from Pap smears to colorectal exams and lung scans—and sharply increasing investments in researching promising new early-detection technologies, particularly blood-based multicancer screening, could conceivably save tens of thousands of lives that we are now losing to failed policies. We have ample evidence proving that treatments and, yes, cures, succeed in vastly greater numbers before the cancerous growths have taken root and spread. We need to act, now, on that medically proven fact.

I am driven by a reality that is too often obscured in public conversations about cancer research and treatment. Despite all that we have learned about the intimate mechanisms of the cell and the stratagems that cancerous mutations use to defeat our cellular level defenses, the rates of death from advanced cancers have hardly changed since the time the government promised a "moonshot" that would end the reign of this disease. I give our doctors enormous credit for making even modest improvements in survival rates, given the brutality of the cancers they are fighting. But, to put it simply, we are asking too much of them if we continue to expect that they can defeat cancer after it has taken hold in the bodies of their patients.

Just look at the historical data. According to the American Cancer Society's annual report on mortality trends, the U.S. cancer death rate peaked in 1991 and has declined since then by around 1.5 percent a year. That represents a 32 percent drop, from 215 deaths per 100,000 people in 1991 to 146 deaths per 100,000 in 2019.[1]

But researchers know that that decline was driven largely by a significant drop in cigarette smoking rates that followed the government's strong antismoking program, bolstered by large-scale mass media campaigns (and increased taxes on cigarettes), which is reducing lung cancer. Remove that factor and, regrettably, the cancer death rates have barely budged.

For example, from 1974 to 1985, 14 percent of patients diagnosed with late-stage colon cancer survived for five years or more,[2] a standard measure of survivability. Patients diagnosed with those cancers between 2011 and 2017 still had a five-year survival rate of 14 percent.[3]

For breast cancer, the five-year survival rate for late-stage illness has gone from 19 percent to 29 percent[4] during that time. For prostate cancer, the five-year survival for late-stage patients was 30 percent between 1974 and 1985 and 31 percent during the 2011 to 2017 period.[5]

FIGURE 1

Survival rates of **late-stage cancers** have remained low and improved very little in forty-plus years.

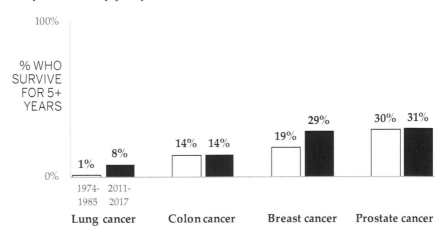

Percentage of patients who were diagnosed with late-stage cancer who survived for five-plus years in the periods 1974–1985 and 2011–2017. Source: American Cancer Society

Just 1 percent of patients with late-stage lung cancer during the 1974 to 1985 window lived five years or more. By 2011 to 2017, that number had risen, but only to 8 percent, certainly a potentially positive result for those with the disease but not a large enough increase to make a dent in the reality that lung cancer remains our most deadly cancer killer, taking roughly 130,000 lives a year.

Even more telling is the flip side of those statistics. Patients diagnosed with early-stage cancers have, in general, benefited from significantly better survival rates.

Between 1974 and 1985, 84 percent of patients with localized, or early-stage, colon cancer survived for five years or more. Between 2011 and 2017, 91 percent did. Early-stage breast cancer survival rates rose to 99 percent, from 91 percent. For prostate cancer, they rose to 99 percent, from 84 percent. Even for lung cancer there was significant improvement, to a 64 percent five-year survival rate from 37 percent.

FIGURE 2

Survival rates of **early-stage cancers** are high and have improved in the last forty-plus years.

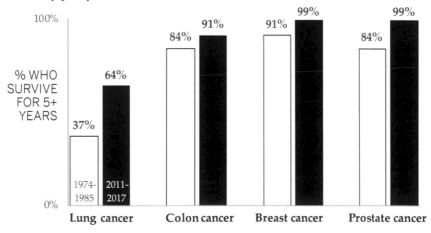

Percentage of patients who were diagnosed with early-stage cancer who survived for 5+ years between 1974–1985 and 2011–2017. Source: American Cancer Society

If you detect and treat cancer early, the odds of survival usually soar. We know how to do that and are developing even better technologies for identifying those cancers in the earliest stages. This is a story that should be more widely understood, even celebrated, and it should inform our cancer priorities and policies.

It is time we shifted our policies to prioritize that truth in our healthcare system, and there should be heavy public spending on media campaigns to educate the public and support the urgency of this new direction. As we make clear in this book, there are substantial hurdles that must be overcome to deliver the results that I believe are possible. Reaching both doctors and patients in large numbers and changing behavior involves administrative, governmental, even societal challenges. Healthcare financial models will have to be adjusted to achieve progress, something we know is too often fought by the industry. But we should be finding ways to screen people before they show symptoms of cancer.

We will show how many of our best screening technologies and techniques have had to struggle for acceptance, how training of technicians needs to be improved, how poor a job we have done in guaranteeing that lower-income communities gain access both to screening and follow-up care. Even with these challenges, we cannot let the perfect be the enemy of the good—we must overcome the problems and issues but not halt the process while we seek refinements.

These are some of the steps we advocate for bringing about this necessary revolution:

We need to redirect more research funding, especially from the huge government sponsors of most medical research, into early-detection technologies, a field with some new and highly promising innovations.

We need to bring underserved, lower-income communities into a new cancer screening system, since a lack of access to health insurance and high-quality care too often relegates these communities to higher rates of late-stage cancers and worse outcomes.

We should fund wider development and use of what are called "patient navigators," trained experts who can guide everyone, step by step, into appropriate screening programs regularly and then, if needed, into treatment.

We need to do a much better job of ensuring that those diagnosed with early-stage cancers receive proper follow-up treatment as promptly as possible so they can enjoy the full benefits of these early-detection technologies.

Significant and sophisticated use of current mass media tools is essential. We need an extensive and well-funded communications and education program to make certain that healthcare providers as well as the generalpublic understand the clear benefits of early-detection screening and how to obtain proper testing on a regular basis.

Consider one success story that demonstrates the positive outcomes that can be achieved when early-detection screening becomes a medical norm. In the first half of the twentieth century, cervical cancer was among the deadliest cancers in women, since it was usually treated only after women developed symptoms, meaning after the disease had advanced. Today, the disease accounts for less than 2 percent of female cancer deaths in the U.S.

WHY? THE PAP SMEAR.

That relatively simple test is the dominant screening procedure for cervical cancer, and it has saved perhaps hundreds of thousands from avoidable early deaths. It detects the presence of even tiny numbers of cancer cells in women who are, generally, asymptomatic, who have no indication that a malignancy has started to grow. Identifying the disease that early allows doctors, in most instances, to defeat it when it is susceptible to a cure.

The Pap smear demonstrates two important issues in the early-detection revolution. First, it shows what is possible. Today, the test is a routine element in most women's healthcare, accepted, understood, and widely employed. But, as we will discuss in a later chapter, it took decades for the test to find acceptance in the medical community, and the implementation was beset for years by a paucity of technicians available to read and interpret the tests, which was largely done by badly overworked, underpaid women.

The Pap smear has arguably done more than any other single in-tervention to cut cancer deaths, but the experience makes clear that implementation is both a crucial and extremely challenging part of the early-detection project.

To help bring about this necessary revolution, there is also the chal-lenge of what does, and does not, excite a sense of human drama. Sav-ing someone teetering on the edge of death from cancer is far more exciting and creates a more compelling narrative than quietly prevent-ing that person from developing a lethal cancer in the first place. So our public conversations too often focus on those dramatic moments, no matter how rare.

Few have articulated this policy challenge better than one of the giants of modern oncology, Bert Vogelstein, a pioneering researcher at the Johns Hopkins Medical School who was one of the first to discern the role of certain genetic mutations in cancer development. Vogelstein is an ardent supporter of placing a greater emphasis on early detection. Our anticancer battle has been "too focused on this idea of retaliation," he said. "Cancers are only incurable once they have spread . . . and in the future we need to focus on detecting them before they have spread."[6]

But human nature loves tales of ingenuity overcoming hurdles. "There's no drama in prevention or preventive medicine. It's much more exciting to develop a new therapy," Vogelstein acknowledged. "When you take a cancer patient and put that patient in remission, even for a few months, that's dramatic. On the other hand, if you prevent all colon cancers, don't expect a ticker-tape parade. No one's going to thank you. There's little excitement in society about the consistent acts that can transform our lives, and this applies to prevention."[7]

It's time we changed the narrative and prepared the way for an early-detection ticker-tape parade. This book explains how we can get there.

Bruce Ratner
Brooklyn, New York
January, 2024

CHAPTER 1
FIGHTING A
LOSING WAR

WHY ARE WE LOSING THE "WAR ON CANCER" SO BADLY?

Our battle against cancer has proven disappointing for many reasons, not the least of which is the basic fact that cancer is a range of diseases that share critical characteristics. It is not one illness with a single set of symptoms or a single set of causes that we are combating. The many different mutations that produce malignancies create different cellular capabilities, different methods for those cells to grow uncontrollably in our organs, to spread throughout the body, and to outsmart our usually efficient defense mechanisms.

This often unstoppable power is due in part to the fact that malignant cancer cells use all of the common biological capabilities of healthy cells, from which they descend, except better. "Cancer cells grow faster, adapt better," Siddhartha Mukherjee, a cancer physician, wrote in his Pulitzer Prize-winning book, *The Emperor of all Maladies: A Biography of Cancer*. "They are more perfect versions of ourselves." They are nurtured and fed by our own bodies, as insiders, not outsiders. The tumors can even grow their own systems of blood vessels to provide sustenance as they expand.

Among the lethal capabilities that the many different types of cancer have in common are that the cells multiply, and mutate, at a far faster rate than healthy cells, accelerating the growth of malignancies. The cancerous DNA is, in other words, corrupted and unstable. Unlike healthy cells, which, in most cases, perform their functions in the body and then die, to be replaced by new healthy cells (or die off if damaged), cancer cells do not die off, at least in those same predictable ways. And cancer cells, unlike healthy human cells, can break free from the sites where they originate, travel through the body and lodge in new organs, where they can renew their malicious attacks.

Because of these complexities, there will never be one "cure," one treatment, or even one means of prevention. The highly publicized "war on cancer," launched by President Richard Nixon in December 1971, is thus not the conventional battle against a single disease that some had envisioned, like the successful earlier fights against small-pox and polio. It is what amounts to an attempt to control a series of intense biological insurgencies involving a constantly shape-shifting enemy in constantly changing battle zones.

"Cancers possessed temperaments, personalities—behaviors," Mukherjee wrote. "And biological heterogeneity demanded therapeutic heterogeneity; the same treatment could not indiscriminately be applied to all." In recognition of this reality, Mukherjee titled a long section of his book "Prevention is the Cure."

In an additional complexity, different cancers have different triggers, different causes. Some cancers are caused by inherited genetic vulnerabilities, passed from parents to their children; some come from behavior that introduces carcinogens, like smoking; some come from environmental factors, such as exposure to asbestos or an overabundance of unfiltered sunlight; and some come from viruses, such as HPV.

And research by Cristian Tomasetti and Bert Vogelstein has suggested that as many as two-thirds of cancers are simply a product of chance, bad luck—a result of tiny mutations that occur randomly in a tiny number of the billions of instances of our healthy cells dividing in the normal course of our lives. Those mutations can then, in a relatively small number of cases, transform the abnormal cells into dangerous malignancies, triggering cancerous growths. In those instances, the disease has no discernible cause; it is just a molecular accident with a potentially lethal outcome.[1]

Thus, determining the exact type of cancer in a patient sometimes requires sophisticated detective work even before treatment options can be considered.

We have also been impeded in our efforts to control cancer by an artificial reality: from the very beginning we've fundamentally misplaced our priorities in fighting the disease. Far too often we fight brutal, rear-guard battles after the cancers have already spread and started to destroy organs. In part, this is by necessity. Doctors often fight diseases only after their patients start exhibiting symptoms.

But, with cancer, there is a better way, which we explain in this book. Immensely important scientific advances in molecular biology and in understanding how healthy cells turn into malignant ones, and then in how they behave, have taught us in an increasing number of cases how to identify the insurgencies in their earliest stages.

Brilliant discoveries by researchers have opened the door to enormously important detection and treatment capabilities. They include ways of detecting biomarkers—telltale biological signs that cancerous cells, even in very small numbers, produce in our bodies. There are promising technologies still in their nascent stages that allow us to find fragments of cancerous DNA that can break free from tumors and get dispersed in the bloodstream.

Some of the most effective screening methods are more straightforward and have been around for decades. In those cases, what we need are intensive programs, supported by professional mass media and social media campaigns, to make primary care physicians as well as patients more aware of the tests. Then we need to make them economical or free for patients, so they become routine, with the necessary medical follow-up built into the programs.

One of the most common tests, Pap smears, involves removing some cells from a woman's cervix and examining them carefully under a microscope. Colonoscopies allow doctors to examine the interior of the colon by threading fine instruments through the bowel that can spot lesions or polyps, which can then be tested to see if they are cancerous. Similarly, low-dose computed tomography, known as LDCT, a type of CT scan, can be used to spot nodules or lesions in lungs.

Early detection benefits from the fact that some cancers take years, even decades to grow into malignant forces rampaging through their hosts. That provides ample time in which they might be detected and treated.

"We have this huge window of opportunity . . . to intervene in that process, to detect those tumors early, and to cure them," said Vogelstein, of the Johns Hopkins University School of Medicine. "But the amount of research that is devoted to these sorts of preventions is essentially trivial compared to that devoted to curing advanced cancers."[2]

The critical breakthrough needed to accelerate progress and sharply reduce cancer mortality rates, a goal very much within reach, is a shift in the policies of government, the medical industry, healthcare insurers, and the public. There must be changes in the types of research we fund, changes in government policy priorities, smarter health insurance coverage for testing and follow-up treatment, and aggressive and enlightened education campaigns to make the public aware of the opportunities and needs for regular cancer screening.

Any effective campaign must also be focused intensively on lower-income and minority communities, which often endure tragically inadequate access to healthcare and health insurance, and thus have historically worse outcomes in fighting cancer compared with more affluent population groups.

This may not be easy, but putting these steps together to accelerate progress could produce one of the most hopeful shifts ever in public health.

Yet there is no sense in denying how much ground we have lost in the battle because of our failure to place an emphasis on early detection. To grasp the problem, it is useful to compare the changing historical mortality rates for cancer, the country's number two killer, with heart disease, the number one killer. The prevalence of heart disease has been declining significantly for years, in large measure because of intensive, well-advertised prevention and good health campaigns, which encourage healthier behavior long before people show symptoms of the disease, as well as rapid intervention when symptoms appear. That stands in stark contrast to how we deal with cancer, where we still fail to reach large portions of the population with screening tests and care.

As a result, the mortality rate for heart disease has plummeted from 588.8 per 100,000 population in 1950 to 257.6 in 2000 and 161.5 in 2019, according to the National Center for Health Statistics. Overall cancer mortality rates, however, rose, then fell, to 199.6 in 2000 and 146.2 in 2019, from 193.9 per 100,000 in 1950. In other words, the once-yawning gap between these two killers has almost disappeared because of stubbornly high cancer mortality.

FIGURE 3

Mortality rates from heart disease have been falling rapidly due to better prevention and detection, while cancer death rates have declined only slightly.

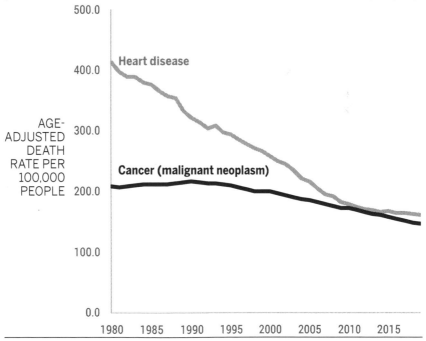

The age-adjusted death rate per 100,000 people for heart disease and cancer.
Source: National Center for Health Statistics

THE MEDICAL DREAM:
TREATING EARLY-STAGE CANCERS

A comprehensive cancer screening campaign would achieve what is, in some respects, the dream of cancer doctors—being able to treat tumors and other malignancies in their nascent stages. The treatment outcomes of those early-stage cancers compared with the outcomes for stage IV cancers is completely lopsided.

Extensive data collected over many decades demonstrate clearly that the survival rates for patients treated for early-stage cancers are, in general, extremely positive. For the years 1974 to 1985, a total of 84 percent of patients with localized, or early-stage colon cancer survived for five years or more. That rose to 91 percent between 2011 and 2017, as a result of improving treatments. For breast cancer, early-stage survival rates rose to 99 percent, from 91 percent, in that same time period. For prostate cancer, they rose to 99 percent, from 84 percent. Patients with early-stage lung cancer, one of the deadliest diseases in its late stages, benefited from a five-year survival rate of 64 percent, up from 37 percent.

The comparable survival rates for patients with late-stage cancers are a fraction of those levels. Better science and even better treatments have not delivered significantly better outcomes in those instances. This just adds emphasis to the reality that once cancer becomes entrenched in the body, this malleable and wily foe is far more challenging to stop.

Yet we continue to place most of our research dollars and research focus on developing medications or technologies for treating those advanced cancers. The European Society for Medical Oncology, a professional organization of cancer doctors, maintains what it calls the Magnitude of Clinical Benefit Scale,[3] a highly detailed, comprehensive compilation of approved cancer drugs scored according to their effectiveness. The database is divided into two sections—one for drug treatments that are potentially curative and the other for those that aren't expected to be curative but that hold out some hope of extending a patient's life.

Of the 366 drug treatment programs currently detailed in the database, just forty-four fit the first category and are regarded as cures. That means the other 322, roughly 90 percent of the list, offer not the possibility of a cure but incremental improvements in survival rates. That is, without doubt, a meaningful benefit for those with cancer and their loved ones, but it would disappoint those who shared the high hopes of President Nixon's call to action in 1971.

Even for the most effective medications, survival gains are almost always measured in months, not years. Take, for instance, the European Society for Medical Oncology's evaluation of Merck's drug Keytruda, which is in a class of medications known as immune system checkpoint inhibitors. It is often used as a treatment for patients with advanced lung cancer as well as some other cancers. Researchers have found that specific proteins on the surface of some cancer cells in effect conceal them from our immune system. That subterfuge protects them from the normal healthy process in which our immune system identifies and kills such intruders. The checkpoint inhibitor drugs cleverly inactivate those specific proteins on the cancer cells and thus make them vulnerable to the body's defenses.

These so-called immunotherapies represent significant breakthroughs, at least in principle, and they have on occasion lived up to expectations, with some late-stage patients experiencing miraculous responses. One famous case is that of President Jimmy Carter, who received Keytruda for metastatic melanoma and survived essentially cancer-free for five years after his diagnosis.

In 2018, a researcher at the MD Anderson Cancer Center in Houston, James P. Allison, and Tasuku Honjo, from Kyoto University in Japan, were jointly awarded the Nobel Prize in Physiology or Medicine for their work illuminating the science underpinning these drugs. Immunotherapies clearly hold great promise.

It is unsurprising, then, that for several indications the European Society for Medical Oncology's drug benefits guide rates Keytruda a 5, the highest score available, indicating a "very high benefit." But what does that score actually mean for most patients? Another five years of life? Four years? Three?

Hardly. According to the study upon which the European Society for Medical Oncology score is based, Keytruda offered advanced lung cancer patients, on a median basis, an extra 9.1 months of survival.[4] Again, that is not insignificant. It is a blessing for many patients and their families. But the early-detection revolution holds the promise of significantly better outcomes.

Most people are in the dark about this reality. In 2012, a team of researchers at Boston's Dana-Farber Cancer Institute set out to learn how well informed late-stage cancer patients really were about the effectiveness of chemotherapy. They surveyed 1,193 patients, 710 with stage IV lung cancer and 483 with stage IV colorectal cancer, asking them whether they thought chemotherapy might cure them. As is the case with the majority of stage IV cancers, both diseases are almost invariably fatal within a relatively brief time, yet 69 percent of lung cancer patients and 81 percent of colorectal cancer patients said they believed that chemotherapy offered them a chance of being cured.[5]

This sort of false hope presents enormous emotional challenges, but it's understandable. Most patients aren't cancer experts, after all. They look for and seize on hopeful signs that they might be able to beat their disease. Doctors and policymakers, on the other hand, are well acquainted with the sobering data on the low survival rates for most advanced cancers. But if you examined how we spend billions in research dollars every year, you would almost certainly come to the opposite conclusion. We need to face this reality head on and discuss significant shifts in our research priorities—not to give up on searching for late-stage treatments, but to place much greater emphasis on the positive success rates for treating early-stage cancers detected through screening methods.

Early detection and cancer treatment development need not be seen as antagonists. On the contrary, earlier detection of cancer improves the outcomes of many drug treatments. The lower a cancer patient's disease burden, the better, on average, they respond to therapy. That's true even for metastatic disease, where chemotherapy cure rates for individuals with micro-metastases (growths too small to be detected on a CT scan) are many times higher than for those with larger metastases.

Earlier detection, in other words, can help some of our so-called miracle drugs come closer to fulfilling their promise. Recent work by a Memorial Sloan-Kettering team led by Luis Diaz Jr., head of the division of solid tumor oncology, and oncologist Andrea Cerek offers a striking example. Using the immunotherapy drug dostarlimab to treat a group of eighteen patients with stage II or stage III colorectal cancer, they achieved full remission in all eighteen individuals—eliminating their tumors without surgery or conventional chemo-radiation therapy, and without worrying complications.[6]

"I believe this is the first time this has happened in the history of cancer," Diaz said.[7]

The study was a small one, and follow-up of these patients is still ongoing, but it demonstrates the potential for early detection and treatments working together. The idea isn't to pit cancer screening against drug development; rather, it's to balance more sensibly our support for the two so that each can work effectively.

Striking that balance has eluded the medical profession for decades. The cancer initiative President Nixon signed in the winter of 1971 called for $400 million to fund the National Cancer Institute, or NCI, in 1972, $500 million in 1973, and $600 million in 1974. Additionally, $20 million was set aside in 1972 for early detection and prevention efforts. That figure rose to $30 million in 1973 and $40 million in 1974.

FIGURE 4

Even with the success of early-detection efforts, support for these strategies make up a tiny percentage of NCI's total funding.

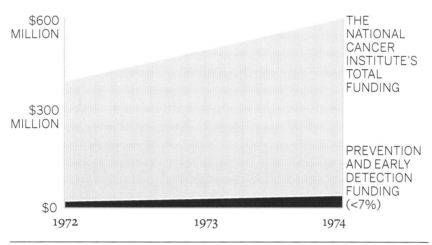

The National Cancer Institute's annual funding 1972–1974. Source: National Cancer Institute

Despite the increased funding for Nixon's "war," prevention and early detection received less than 7 percent of the spending, and that figure has barely budged. In 2021,[8] the NCI spent just 9 percent of its $6.4 billion budget on detection and diagnosis. That compares to 16 percent for basic cancer biology, 24 percent spent on treatments research, and 21 percent on cancer causation studies.

As of April 2022, the NCI had ninety-four ongoing clinical trials evaluating different cancer screening methods, a number of which are not focused on early detection but instead on areas like detection of recurrence in cancer patients following treatment. By contrast, it had 4,830 trials looking into cancer therapies.

Other organizations support cancer research, and some are more focused on early detection—such as the Prevent Cancer Foundation—but the NCI is far and away the largest source of cancer research dollars in the U.S. Consider that in 2021, the Centers for Disease Control and Prevention, or CDC, a major government hub for cancer screening, called for a total of $381 million for cancer prevention and control,[9] not all of which went toward screening programs. The American Cancer Society, the country's largest private, nonprofit cancer research funder, spends slightly less than $60 million per year on screening and treatment combined, roughly 10 percent of its overall budget.[10] Taken together, that's still short of the meager slice of NCI's research budget allocated to detection and diagnosis. The NCI dominates the U.S. cancer research landscape, and it thus plays an outsized role in establishing priorities.

BASIC SCIENCE VS. CLINICAL APPLICATIONS

Research priorities are influenced, of course, by the protean, clever, and deceptive strategies employed by cancer cells. The medical profession has, from the start, placed an emphasis on answering important questions about cancer's causes, how it works at the cellular level, why some people fight it better than others.

Basic science, in other words. The people who run the NCI and have run it historically "are people who really believe in biology," said Karen Emmons, a professor at Harvard's T.H. Chan School of Public Health. "They are largely bench scientists. And that is certainly important, but when you look at how the resources are spent, there is a bias."

It's a bias that predates the 1971 start of the war on cancer and that was, in fact, an important factor in shaping the debate leading up to its launch. In his 1977 book on the history of the war, *Cancer Crusade: The Story of the National Cancer Act of 1971*, social scientist Richard A. Rettig details how the battle over the legislation was defined by the long-running dispute within the research community over whether more emphasis should be placed on finding treatments or exploring the basic biology behind cancer (in the hope that that knowledge would eventually lead to new treatments).

The question at that time was whether scientific knowledge about cancer had advanced to the point where it made sense to push for clinical applications, or whether it remained so mysterious a disease that more basic research had to come first. This debate was reflected in the narrower question of whether the NCI should be broken out as a separate government organization, distinct from the National Institutes of Health, the NIH, or whether it should remain one among many other institutes within the NIH.

Broadly speaking, advocates of an independent NCI promoted a more applied, clinical emphasis for cancer research. They wanted to focus on drugs and treatments first. Their opponents, on the other hand, insisted that continued focus on the fundamental science of cancer was the better approach for delivering more effective treatments later. They argued that researchers pursuing basic science would benefit from close interaction with the other NIH divisions and so should remain a part of the institute.

The latter group, which comprised much of the medical research establishment, was additionally (some might say primarily) concerned that an independent NCI would drain funding from the broader NIH system, leaving less money on the table for noncancer scientists.

Of course, there was a political angle, as well. In late 1970, Senator Edward M. Kennedy took over as chair of the health subcommittee of the Senate Committee on Labor and Public Welfare. Kennedy planned to introduce in early 1971 the Conquest of Cancer Act, which called for an increase in cancer research funding and the creation of an independent organization, the National Cancer Authority, that would replace NCI and function outside the NIH's control.

The political calculations then took over. The Nixon administration considered Kennedy a potential challenger in the 1972 election and so moved to undercut his leadership on the cancer battle, which the administration viewed as a popular issue. In January 1971, Nixon used his State of the Union address to preempt Kennedy's bill, announcing that he planned to call "for an appropriation of an extra $100 million to launch an intensive campaign to find a cure for cancer." The following week, Nixon released his 1972 budget, which included the first $100 million commitment along with an additional $232 million in funding for the NCI.

Unlike Kennedy, Nixon didn't move to separate NCI from the NIH, distinguishing his effort from the Senate bill. When Kennedy held three days of hearings on the bill in March 1971, this distinction was central to the debate. In the end, the Nixon administration won. The NCI remained part of the NIH, marking a victory for the basic research crowd, an orientation that continues to shape the institute and its priorities. It helped that the basic research priority was supported by nearly every medical science group in the country. The American Cancer Society was one of the few organizations that signed on to Kennedy's vision.

APPLYING EARLY-DETECTION STRATEGIES MORE EQUITABLY

But while Nixon, Kennedy, and their compatriots battled over the direction cancer research would take, another, seemingly separate, concern occasionally entered the debate. Testifying before the Senate committee in March 1971, Sidney Farber, a pioneer of chemotherapy and a giant of cancer research, told legislators that in "the place we have reached today, one-third of all patients are being cured of cancer and it would be possible to cure one-half of all patients with cancer if we could apply for the benefit of every patient of the country the knowledge and early diagnosis and treatment which is available in centers of expertise."[11]

Speaking later during that same congressional session, Senator Hubert Humphrey echoed and sharpened Farber's message.

"If all our citizens could receive the same quality of diagnosis and treatment now available at the best treatment centers, we could significantly reduce the death rate from cancer," he said. "This calls for no great scientific breakthrough . . . this simply calls for a more equitable, just distribution of the resources already available to the more privileged members of our society."[12]

Kennedy himself made the same point during the hearings, adding the observation that, even in 1971, none of this was news.

"As long ago as 1965," he said, "eminent scientists and physicians in the cancer field testified that if we could only fully apply all that was then known, we could have saved many persons whose lives were lost to cancer."[13]

If we could only fully apply all that was then known . . .

Here was a collection of scientists, advocates, doctors, and administrators representing the full spectrum of the American healthcare establishment, gathering with congressional leaders to map out how billions of dollars in new cancer research funding would be spent. Numerous authoritative voices declared that a critical part of the problem was that the establishment was failing to apply known, highly effective approaches already in hand.

But the two sides were not listening to each other, or to the experts. Each side—Nixon's proponents of basic science and Kennedy's advocates of expanded clinical work—shared the same basic premise: new knowledge, new science was required to make progress against cancer. More research in all areas was needed, but significant progress could have been achieved with the tools that were at hand. As Senator Humphrey declared, "This calls for no great scientific breakthrough . . . this simply calls for a more equitable, just distribution of the resources already available."

This remains true today. Early detection and equitable treatment have the potential to dramatically cut cancer mortality right now. The four leading cancer killers—lung, colorectal, breast, and prostate—account for nearly half of U.S. cancer deaths. Effective screening methods exist for all of them. Those methods are not only underused, but their application is inconsistent. The profession doesn't screen vast numbers of people who absolutely should be tested—the poor, the underinsured, and those who have trouble accessing the healthcare system for reasons of language, education, or geography. The evidence also shows that when doctors do conduct early-detection tests, they sometimes do it poorly. And then there is the related issue: even when a properly administered screening test does find an early-stage cancer, too often patients fail to receive appropriate care. Proper follow-up treatment for those discovered to have cancers is an essential piece of the necessary revolution.

What good is more research if we don't apply what we learn?

Between 2002 and 2010, the NCI spent $250 million and untold work hours on a trial investigating whether low-dose computed tomography, or LDCT, a promising new type of CT scan, could reduce lung cancer deaths by detecting tumors early. It turned out that it could—a result with tremendous implications for fighting the leading cause of cancer deaths worldwide.

More than a decade later, despite that breakthrough, only 4.5 percent of patients who should be screened for lung cancer are getting the scans.[14] From a scientific standpoint, the NCI trial, known as the National Lung Screening Trial, was a success, demonstrating the clear value of lung cancer screening. But the real-world application of this technology has been modest. Too few who are at risk get the test. Without that application, the effort—the largest and most expensive randomized controlled trial for a screening test in U.S. history—will be remembered as, essentially, a waste.

There should be well-organized media and social media information campaigns to make the public aware of these screening technologies and there should be incentives to encourage expanded adoption. It should be emphasized that such campaigns are needed because, as this book will explain, the rollout of even the best early-detection methods have faced frustrating roadblocks and resistance. That simply should not be the case.

Colorectal cancer screening is one of the most effective anticancer measures in existence. But application of the gold standard procedure, the colonoscopy, varies wildly throughout the country. (Other tests exist that use stool or blood samples for colorectal cancer screening, though these are generally not as effective at picking up early-stage and precancerous lesions.)

In 2018, researchers from the CDC published a study looking at colorectal cancer screening by county. The screening rates ranged from as low as 40 percent in some parts of Alaska to as high as 80 percent in parts of Florida.[15] The average nationwide was 67 percent, with only thirty-one of the 3,142 counties in the U.S. reporting screening rates of 75 percent or higher. That should be a floor, not a ceiling.

Researchers surveyed mammography usage, a key test for breast cancer, in a separate paper published in 2018 that arrived at similar findings. While mammogram rates were generally found to be higher than rates for colorectal cancer screening (78 percent of women were up to date with their mammograms), they also varied tremendously, ranging from a low of 69 percent in Idaho to a high of almost 90 percent in Massachusetts.[16]

Johns Hopkins's Vogelstein may have been right that preventive measures lack the drama of late-stage medical cures, and thus they fail to seize the public's imagination. That's human nature, but it can make for terrible public policy.

IMPLEMENTATION BLIND SPOTS

In 2005, researchers at Virginia Commonwealth University published a paper describing what they called "the break-even point," the point at which it becomes more beneficial to focus on expanding the implementation of a successful type of medical intervention rather than spending money on improving it or finding a new one.[17]

Frequently, they wrote, "technological advances must yield dramatic, often unrealistic increases in efficacy to do more good" than could be achieved simply by applying the older practices or technologies more broadly.

The case of lung cancer screening illustrates this perfectly. The NCI's National Lung Screening Trial found that LDCT screening reduced lung cancer mortality by 20 percent. This figure has been the subject of debate, with some experts arguing that, in fact, a poorly designed trial badly understated the benefits, which may be well over 50 percent. In one sense, it's obviously important to understand, using such trials, exactly how many lives would be saved by the effective application of LDCT screening. But so long as only 4.5 percent of the eligible at-risk population is being screened, the test has only a modest impact on the terrible and continuing impact of lung cancer. That underscores the significance of the often-underappreciated importance of the implementation element of the early-detection revolution.

Our blindness to these simple facts extends to other areas of health-related spending priorities. While we put tens of billions of dollars each year toward medical research, we spend a small fraction of that studying specifically how to apply new treatments and procedures to the appropriate populations. How useful is our knowledge if we do not find ways to use it to produce a healthier population and better outcomes?

The federal agency primarily responsible for this kind of research, the Agency for Healthcare Research and Quality, has a budget that typically ranges from $350 million to $450 million. The NIH's budget in 2021 was $43 billion. In other words, for every dollar spent pursuing new science, we spent roughly one cent working out how to best use it—and only a fraction of that was devoted to research into spreading the benefits of early detection of cancer.

Lack of funding is a constant challenge. Several years ago, researchers from Washington University in St. Louis surveyed state and local health departments to learn how many of them had been forced to terminate effective cancer screening and prevention programs due to lack of funding or other factors. The answer? A depressing 28 percent.[18]

One of the saddest aspects of this inattention is the failure to ensure that patients who do receive screening and are found to have early forms of cancer get needed treatment. In one example, an analysis of Medicaid billing records for residents of Washington, D.C., in 2017 and 2018 found that only 47 percent of the patients on Medicaid who had been diagnosed with cancer were receiving medical care for their condition.

Why do we allow this to happen?

"I would say that's the million-dollar question, but it's really more like hundreds of billions of dollars if you add up what we've spent [fighting cancer]," said Ross Brownson, one of the researchers on the Washington University study and a professor of public health at the university. Brownson is a leading figure in what has become known as implementation science—the study of how people put innovations and scientific discoveries into practice.

"The reasons are in some ways societal," he suggested. "Policymakers tend to be reactive, and when they are reacting, they are often reacting to a crisis or something that is deemed to have a lot of immediacy. Early detection is kind of a long slog. It's not, oh, I'll do this now and in the next few months we're going to see a lowering in the rate of breast cancer or the lowering of the rate of colon cancer."

Today, the opportunities in effective implementation are more urgent than ever, because we're standing on the verge of what could be transformational advances in the early detection of cancer. Tools like genomic sequencing—determining the complete set of genetic material in a cell's DNA—have opened new approaches that could augment current screening procedures and enable new types of early detection of cancers. These technologies could help us test for cancers that cannot now be detected in the earliest stages, including the promise of blood-based tests that could potentially screen for fifty or more cancers with one blood draw. Just as critical as the task of refining such technologies is the uphill battle to deploy them widely and wisely.

This runs contrary to a popular notion that once an innovative scientist develops a useful invention the hard work is done. Implementation may seem mundane, by contrast, but it also requires large amounts of creativity and persistence.

None of this is to deny the importance of technological and scientific advances or the need to invest in basic research. Innovation has been essential to what gains we have made in the fight against cancer and will help drive progress in the years to come. Equally essential, though, is that we pay careful attention to the screening tools that we already have, to the possibilities enabled by past discoveries.

Science fiction author William Gibson is said to have once commented that "the future is already here—it's just not very evenly distributed." That is often cited as an expression of the idea that in many ways we've made more progress than many appreciate because they have yet to experience it themselves.

The observation also underscores the more discouraging reality that the fruits of our knowledge, our greatest intellectual insights, and especially our powerful medical capabilities, have not reached everyone that could or should benefit. That is an apt perspective on the current landscape of early detection and treatment of cancer—and should serve as a clarion call for urgent remedial action.

CHAPTER 2
SOLVING THE IMPLEMENTATION PUZZLE:
DECADES OF DELAYS IN THE BATTLE AGAINST CERVICAL CANCER

AT AN AMERICAN CANCER SOCIETY CONFERENCE IN 1969, Charles Cameron, the organization's medical and scientific director, described to an audience the "two most striking changes" then appearing in epidemiological surveys of cancer.[1] In a sort of split-screen snapshot, he first highlighted data showing alarming increases in the incidence of and deaths from lung cancer, a result, of course, of the steep increases in smoking rates in the U.S., beginning in the 1930s and 1940s. Cameron then shared equally dramatic but positive news: deaths from cervical cancer were plummeting. It had been among the deadliest types of cancer in women in the early years of the twentieth century, but by the time of his speech the death rate had been cut by more than half and was still falling. Today, the disease accounts for less than 2 percent of female cancer deaths in the U.S.

The decline was almost entirely attributable to one of the great success stories in the history of cancer treatment—widespread uptake of an effective early-detection test, the Pap smear. It is a model of the immense power of such screening strategies in saving lives. It is also, however, a sobering lesson in the daunting challenges early-detection tests can face in being accepted and used in large population groups, no matter how promising.

The Pap smear was the first cancer screening technology to be used on a large proportion of the population, yet it struggled for acceptance by doctors and patients, and took decades before it was widely available. The test's bumpy history illustrates the surprising rigidities that can get in the way of deploying new cancer screening tools.

The Pap smear was developed in the 1920s by a Greek doctor, George Papanicolaou, who observed that it was possible to distinguish between healthy and cancerous cervical cells by examining them under a microscope.[2] That was not his original intention. He was studying the female reproductive cycle and took samples of women's vaginal cells in an effort to, among other things, diagnose pregnancies. The samples were spread as "smears" on slides under the microscope for closer examination. Through the research, he began to realize that he could, in some instances, discern the presence of unhealthy malignant cells among the healthy ones, and that these were telltale early signs of cancer.

One of the most promising aspects of this discovery was that Papanicolaou determined that he could spot these troubling malignant cells even before the women had developed symptoms of cancer. This represented a leap ahead in treatment, because by the time women had become symptomatic their cancers had usually spread and were extremely difficult to stop.

Trained as a doctor and zoologist in Greece and Germany, Papanicolaou had immigrated with his wife, Mary, to the United States in 1913 hoping to obtain a research position at an American institution. It was a struggle for a newcomer. He worked briefly as a rug salesman at Gimbels Department Store before he managed to secure a part-time job as an assistant in the Department of Pathology and Bacteriology at New York Hospital. His boss, the physician William Elser, recognized his talents quickly and recommended Papanicolaou for a position at Cornell University Medical College (now Weill Cornell Medicine) where he would spend the next forty-seven years and perform essentially all his important work.[3]

Once he discovered and proved the efficacy of his early-detection technique, he made a first presentation of his findings in January 1928, at what was called the Proceedings of the Third Race Betterment Conference. It was the last in a series of meetings held by the Race Betterment Foundation, a eugenics organization founded by American cereal magnate John Harvey Kellogg,[4] a physician who openly embraced a racist philosophy of protecting whites against racial mixing and "degeneracy."

"THE MALIGNANT TUMOR CELL HAS NOTHING ABSOLUTELY CHARACTERISTIC . . ."

For Papanicolaou, it was an inauspicious debut, and not only because of the forum in which it took place. His fellow physicians were unconvinced that the approach was either feasible or necessary. There was also skepticism among pathologists that cytology—examining groups of cells—could be used to diagnose cancer. A comment made by German pathologist Max Borst the same year as Papanicolaou's presentation summed up established opinion at the time:

"... the malignant tumor cell has nothing absolutely characteristic, neither in respect to morphology nor chemically or by any other quality."[5]

It didn't help that the report of Papanicolaou's discovery, published in the conference proceedings, was marred by typos ("cancerous" was misspelled as "conscious" multiple times) and poorly printed photographs.[6] Following the conference, Papanicolaou largely dropped the idea and returned to studying the female reproductive issues that had first motivated his research.

More than a decade passed before he again focused on detecting cancers. In 1939, Joseph Hinsey took over as chair of the departments of Anatomy and Physiology at the Cornell University Medical College. Reviewing his staff's research, Hinsey came across Papanicolaou's report from the 1928 conference and encouraged him to return to the idea. He promised financial support and helped Papanicolaou establish a collaboration with H. F. Traut, a gynecological pathologist at Cornell who could provide him with the patient samples he needed to further refine and validate the method for identifying cancer cells in the "smears." From that point on, vaginal smears were taken from every woman admitted to New York Hospital for gynecological attention and were sent to Papanicolaou's lab for analysis.[7] The pace of study and proof accelerated.

In March 1941, Papanicolaou and Traut presented a study of their findings to the New York Obstetrical Society. In August, it was published in the *American Journal of Obstetrics and Gynecology*. The same year, the Commonwealth Fund, a philanthropy, provided an $1,800 grant to support Papanicolaou's ongoing research, the first of $124,000 in funding—a significant sum in those days, the equivalent of nearly $2.5 million today—it would provide over the next decade.[8]

Papanicolaou and his colleagues demonstrated in large cohorts of women that cytological examination of vaginal smears—what would eventually come to be known as Pap smears, after its inventor—could detect cervical cancer in asymptomatic women and detect it before it was apparent in biopsies or had become invasive. That was the great power of this test; it caught the disease at an early stage when there was a very good chance the patient could be treated and the cancer stopped.

The test was able to do even better than that. Cancer is classified into different numbered stages, with the higher stages designating more severe forms of the disease. Stage I cancers are generally small and still confined to one area within the patient's tissue. Stage II and III cancers have spread into surrounding tissue and the lymph nodes. Stage IV disease, also known as metastatic cancer, has spread in more areas of the patient's body and is present in different organs.

There is also something called stage 0 cancer, which, as the name implies, isn't really cancer at all. Also known as carcinoma in situ, stage 0 is the term for abnormal cells that have started on a path of mutation that could eventually turn malignant. Dysplasia is another term used to describe the presence of these abnormal cells.

The Pap smear can identify these precancerous cells as well as those that have already been transformed into malignancies. The test allows doctors to identify and remove those suspicious cells in their precancerous states.

By the late 1940s, the Pap smear's proven capabilities had finally won over many doctors and well-known medical institutes and health-care organizations, perhaps the most important being the recently launched American Cancer Society (ACS). The organization had been founded in 1945 as a successor to the American Society for the Control of Cancer, which had been dedicated to helping women identify and seek treatment for uterine cancer. In 1948, the ACS held the First National Cytology Conference, where the Pap smear was featured prominently.[9] It had taken two decades, but Papanicolaou's early-detection test had at last been embraced by the medical community.

It may have felt like Papanicolaou and his colleagues and supporters could finally enjoy the achievement of reaching this remarkable scientific summit, but the trek was far from over—an indication of how trying the struggles over early-detection methods can be. There were other Everests they had to climb to bring the test to the wider public.

When Papanicolaou first started to describe his method, the idea of finding and treating a carcinoma in situ was a relatively novel concept for most doctors. There was little understanding of how common such abnormalities were as precursors to full-blown cervical cancer. Even as knowledge of these potentially dangerous cells spread in the 1940s, the concerns were initially accepted mostly by gynecologists and others working outside traditional pathology departments. That made it difficult for many primary care doctors to know exactly what they were looking for and if interventions were needed.

Even more challenging was this perplexing reality: researchers did not know exactly which abnormal cells or what proportion of precancerous cases would end up advancing into cervical cancers. These were complicated medical questions with serious implications. Studies throughout the 1940s and 1950s established that a substantial percentage of women with such abnormal cells—called cervical hyperplasia—went on to develop invasive cancer. But scientists were unable to identify any specific characteristics that distinguished the hyperplasic cells that would progress into threatening malignancies from those that would not.

That was an immensely important riddle for doctors to solve because treatment in those days often meant a radical hysterectomy or radiation, both of which involved serious side effects, including infertility. Doctors faced the risk of harming their patients without knowing if it was necessary to save their lives or if it amounted to a dangerous overreaction. Since then, researchers have developed more targeted procedures like cone biopsies and laser ablation surgeries that remove only the precancerous cells while leaving the rest of the uterus intact. Those procedures can also preserve a women's fertility and give patients and doctors more treatment options.

But determining which precancerous cells justify harsher treatments and which do not remains a problem. It is still one of the major difficulties facing early detection of cancer, an example of the challenges medical science faces in unraveling the inner mysteries of our cells.

THE SCIENCE WAS READY FOR PAP SMEARS, BUT WERE DOCTORS?

Another problem that the pioneers of Pap smear testing confronted was ensuring that there were enough technicians and specialists trained to conduct the exams properly. This prompted Papanicolaou and his supporters to warn initially against too rapid a rollout of the screening program.[10] Most pathologists didn't have the cytologic expertise required to interpret Pap smears with the necessary high level of accuracy. A national screening campaign would generate millions of samples needing confident examination and analysis. Advertising Pap smears widely before enough pathologists had been trained could undermine the entire effort.

Papanicolaou had expected this problem. In the years before the 1948 cytology conference, he had hosted pathologists in his lab and instructed them in cytology and the interpretation of vaginal smears. In 1947, he had launched a formal course in cytology, inviting seventy participants, including forty-five pathologists from different regions of the country.[11]

Papanicolaou was right to be concerned about problems in the rollout of the Pap smear on a broader scale. In coming years, the Pap smear would require various technical refinements in response to new evidence and would encounter challenges to its accuracy, including false positives and false negatives, misdiagnoses, and ambiguous readings. (False positives—believing that a test has detected a cancerous growth when, in fact, there is none—is a constant concern with screening tests that we discuss in detail in other chapters.) But the seemingly straightforward matter of having enough trained personnel would remain one of the most pressing initial problems.

Throughout the 1950s, research sites around the country launched studies of the Pap smear, testing the technique in hundreds of thousands of women in order to collect large pools of data on its effectiveness. A report from a 1959 Department of Defense appropriations hearing provided a review of these efforts, detailing the structure of each trial and the different clinical questions being explored. The report observed that "there is a tremendous shortage of trained personnel . . . in the entire field of cytology."[12]

Technicians needed to have sufficient training to be able to independently examine specimens and determine if abnormal or cancerous cells were present, a task, the report added, that "requires a considerable amount of judgment and involves a certain degree of responsibility."

Given the amount of education and training required, recruiting and retaining cytology technicians was "extremely difficult." The report added that most of these technicians were "young women of marriageable age who stay in the field for only a limited period of time."

The report also detailed steps the National Cancer Institute was taking to address this shortfall. These included a trainee program where technicians were given on-the-job training at cytology projects then run by the NCI. Additionally, the NCI allocated $100,000 in 1958 and 1959 to train roughly thirty cytology technicians and sixty pathologists. Given the NCI's budget of more than $75 million in 1959,[13] that was a modest investment for such a promising test.

The unmet demand for well-trained technicians was acute in part because the task was so difficult and time-consuming. Papanicolaou himself once told a colleague that he could take as long as half an hour to read particularly difficult slides, a big commitment when there are large backlogs of smears to examine.

By their nature, Pap smears rely less on any technological wizardry than on human judgment. During the procedure, a medical professional uses a brush or a special spatula to scrape cells from a woman's cervix. These cells are spread across a microscope slide then fixed (a chemical process that preserves the cells) and stained to enable easier identification of important cellular features and abnormalities. The smear typically contains several hundred thousand cells, which must be carefully examined by the cytology technician.

The technician will usually begin at relatively low magnifying power, allowing them to move quickly across the slide. They switch to a higher resolution when they need to investigate potential abnormalities. On average, reading a slide takes an experienced technician five to ten minutes, but that five to ten minutes requires careful, sustained concentration. Any abnormal cells are then reviewed by a pathologist for clearer identification.

50 CENTS A SLIDE

Market economics suggest that the simple solution to the shortage of technicians should have been an increase in wages to attract more entrants to the field. But that never happened. The job was a low-paying, high-stress, female-dominated occupation, according to sociologists Monica Casper and Adele Clarke. It took advantage of the narrow job options women faced in those years to pay them poorly in return for their expertise, in spite of the lifesaving promise of offering the Pap smear at scale.[14]

Carol Carriere, a cytologist, recalled for an article in the journal *Laboratory Medicine* that, during her start in the field in the early 1970s, some technicians she knew were being paid 50 cents per slide and "working two or three jobs to make a decent wage."[15]

"I heard rumors of cytotechnologists reading 200 to 300 slides per day," she said. Assuming an eight-hour workday, that amounts to two minutes per slide, or less, and that's without any breaks—an impossible pace to sustain while maintaining acceptable standards of accuracy and quality.

In a field where the margin for error can mean lives needlessly lost, that is a troubling record. Even under good conditions, technicians miss cervical abnormalities between 10 percent and 20 percent of the time.[16] Cervical cancer often takes a decade or more to develop, and women are urged to get Pap smear testing done regularly, sometimes annually or every few years. That gives doctors multiple opportunities to catch the disease early in its development and to take preventive steps, at least in theory.

Even so, the poor laboratory practices Carriere described may have cost some women their lives. Around the same time that she started her cytology career, federal officials investigated a lab that had a contract to read Pap smears for the Air Force. According to a record of the examination by a pathologist, William Frable, seven women whose Pap smears were analyzed by that lab later died of cervical cancer.[17] Similar incidents occurred at labs throughout the country.

There were also reports of some labs offering Pap smear testing as a loss leader. They would charge well below cost as a way of encouraging the doctors to send them additional, more lucrative lab work. The physicians reportedly could pay the lab its artificially low rate, then bill patients or insurers for the true cost of the tests. Insurers and the government have since cracked down on these so-called pass-through billing practices, but such arrangements incentivized laboratories to put volume over quality, compromising the accuracy of the readings from the Pap smears.

Activist groups like the San Francisco-based Coalition for the Medical Rights of Women began drawing attention to the problem of high Pap smear error rates. News reports in national and local publications also brought awareness of the issue to a broader audience. According to the journal article by Casper and Clarke, these stories included reports of "High false negative rates resulting in personal tragedies, oppressive working conditions for cytotechnologists, high profit margins for poor quality work, unregulated 'Pap mill' laboratories with inadequately trained and unlicensed staff."[18]

A series of articles in 1987 by *Wall Street Journal* investigative reporter Walter Bogdanich hit the business particularly hard. Bogdanich detailed the travails of overworked cytology technicians and patients affected by sloppy Pap smear readings. The pieces sparked outrage and encouraged Congress to hold hearings on allegations of fraud and malpractice in the clinical labs. They also won Bogdanich a well-deserved Pulitzer Prize.

CONGRESS TAKES OVER

Those hearings came sixty years after Papanicolaou's introduction of the Pap smear at the Third Race Betterment conference and forty years after the ACS's First National Cytology Conference, which provided proof of the promise of this early-detection screening. Despite the decades that had passed, offering the medical profession opportunities to refine the tests and spread their benefits equitably, the hearings painted an unflattering picture of cervical cancer screening and its checkered track record. Some specialists in the field were appalled and open in their criticism.

"If your wife, daughter, or mother had a Pap smear within the last year, the cells in that Pap smear were initially evaluated under a microscope by a cytotechnologist," Shirley Greening, a professor of cytotechnology and cytogenetics at Thomas Jefferson University in Philadelphia, said in her testimony at the hearing. "I am here today to tell you that her doctor may not have taken the time or known how to collect an adequate Pap smear; that the laboratory where her Pap smear was sent may not be of the quality or caliber that you or your relative assumed; that the technologist reading that Pap smear was too tired because of overwork to make an accurate diagnosis on the Pap smear; that the pathologist who could have reviewed her Pap smear may not have been specially trained to do so; and that the report that was sent back to her doctor may not have been written in words that her doctor understands; and that if there was something wrong with her Pap smear, we might not know until it is too late because now or in the near future she might have cervical cancer."[19]

Greening went on to detail what Bogdanich and others had described in their reporting on the industry: how competition among labs had led some to position Pap smears as a loss leader; how this had led to even more overwork of cytology technicians, with some reading 200 to 300 slides per day for as little as 50 cents per slide; how some labs incentivized technicians to read slides even more quickly by offering bonuses for each slide that they examined above their daily quota; how some labs, in violation of Medicare regulations, encouraged technicians to take slides home after work to read; how labs often cut corners on their quality control processes in order to keep costs as low as possible; how fast-paced production was prioritized "at the expense of diagnostic accuracy."

Malfeasance and slipshod practices were not the only problems highlighted at the hearings. The technician shortage that Papanicolaou identified decades before had persisted. If anything, it was getting worse. According to testimony provided by the American Society for Cytotechnology, low salaries and overwork had driven many technicians from the field. The organization cited the example of a technician who had recently left her job, explaining that she could make "$15,000 more as a lousy computer programmer than she did as a good cytotechnologist."[20]

The society said that the cytology business's reliance on women, who had accepted lower pay because of employment barriers in other industries, was under pressure as well. "The entry pool into the profession is also declining because traditional female barriers to other more lucrative job opportunities are breaking down," the cytotechnology society said.

Exacerbating the shortage was the fact that the number of training programs for cytologists had plummeted, to 39 in 1988, from 110 in the early 1970s. And only about 65 percent of the available student slots at the programs were filled. The society estimated that about 130 trained cytology technicians would enter the workforce in 1988, drastically short of the 400 open positions.

What makes the story of cytology technicians so unfortunate, and instructive, is not that they sometimes made mistakes—human error will always play a role in such procedures—but that the healthcare system, in effect, encouraged those mistakes by building systems that emphasized haste and high profitability over accuracy.

THE HPV BREAKTHROUGH

A number of scientific refinements and breakthroughs have since played an important role in improving prevention and early detection of cervical cancer. In the late 1990s, so-called thin layer cell collection technologies that enabled more thorough sampling of a woman's cervical cells were rolled out. Highly accurate, automated scanning instruments were introduced around the same time. These devices are able to read Pap smear slides and, in some cases, even rule out cervical abnormalities without any human intervention, helping to lift some of the laborious workload from the cytology technicians.

In a highly significant advance, scientists in the 1980s uncovered the causal link between human papillomavirus infections, HPV, and cervical cancer. That has opened important new avenues for prevention of the disease. Doctors can prioritize HPV-positive women for more intensive regular screening. Some newer guidelines recommend screening using HPV testing alone, which some studies have shown may be more accurate than Pap smears.[21] The development of HPV vaccines has also provided a new tool for combating cervical cancer, allowing doctors to prevent the infections that, scientists now know, are a primary cause of the disease.

Since HPV vaccines were introduced in the U.S. in 2006, infection rates among young women have declined by more than 80 percent,[22] raising the realistic prospect that the medical field could potentially eliminate most instances of cervical cancer, an extraordinary lifesaving development.

In 1988, several months after the congressional hearings where Shirley Greening and others told their depressing stories of poorly run labs and weak testing accuracy, the federal government issued the Clinical Laboratory Improvement Amendments, a package of standards that strengthened federal regulation of clinical laboratories and capped the number of slides a technician could review at 100 per day. The standards also established quality control measures for testing laboratories.

Governments started to address the pass-through billing practices that contributed to the Pap smear's problems. A number of states and private insurers tightened standards for billing, prohibiting the most abusive practices.

There are many things we still don't know about this dangerous disease. Like most cancers, it seems to have an ability to stay one step ahead of our defenses, with some patients. We do know, though, how to train cytology technicians. We do know how to clamp down on abusive billing arrangements that create improper incentives. We do know how to regulate labs to limit the burden placed on overworked technicians.

THE PAP SMEAR

1913 — George Papanicolaou, a Greek doctor, immigrates to the U.S.

1928 — Papanicolaou authors paper saying in examining a small "smear" of cervical cells under a microscope he can identify cancer in early stage. Colleagues are skeptical so he drops research.

1939 — With new encouragement, Papanicolaou revisits his research on finding early cancers in cervical "smears."

1941 — Papanicolaou's success in proving his discovery leads to naming the procedure the "Pap smear."

1947 — Papanicolaou teaches course on how to use Pap smears for early detection.

1948 — Pap smears cancer screening technique accepted by medical experts.

1959 — NCI invests $100k in training cytology technicians to analyze smears for cancer. As more testing sites open, experts report large shortage of trained technicians.

1969 — Data show cervical cancer deaths have been cut by more than half and continue to decline as use of Pap smears spreads.

1987 — Investigative reporter Walter Bogdanich identifies poor testing and overwork of underpaid technicians in Pap smear labs.

1988 — There is critical shortage of cytology technicians and steep decline in training programs. Congress passes Clinical Laboratory Improvement Amendments to establish quality control in Pap smear testing labs.

2006 — Vaccine for HPV, a cause of cervical cancer, are introduced and infection rates decline by 80%.

The story of the Pap smear is a medical journey involving inspiring, even heroic breakthroughs—but it is also a tale of missed warning signs, inattention, shortsighted practices, and misguided priorities. It represented a powerful medical opportunity that the profession almost missed, which even its ultimate success cannot paper over. But it has ultimately been a critical lifesaver, a milestone in the story of screening tests, and a powerful affirmation of the necessity of reorienting cancer policies around early detection.

What has it taught the medical field? A look at early-detection efforts for the deadliest cancer of all, lung cancer, offers another illustrative story.

CHAPTER 3

HAVE WE BOTCHED A LIFESAVING LUNG CANCER SCREENING TEST?

ON A SUMMER WEEKEND IN 1999, CHRISTINE BERG WAS vacationing at a friend's beach house in Delaware when she received a surprise phone call from Richard Klausner, a colleague who led the National Cancer Institute, the NCI. Researchers at Weill Cornell Medicine had just published a study in *The Lancet*, the medical journal, he said, with data that suggested a diagnostic technology called low-dose computed tomography, or LDCT, could prove a powerful new lung cancer screening tool.[1]

The advance was amplified further by *The New York Times*, which published a follow-up article that quoted one leader of the study, Claudia Henschke, saying that, by spotting malignant growths in their earliest stages, the LDCT screening might potentially increase lung cancer survival rates, then 15 percent, to 80 percent.[2] If correct, the data suggested they had achieved a momentous breakthrough that could save perhaps tens of thousands a year from succumbing to preventable early deaths from the most lethal of all cancers.

The issue was urgent enough that Klausner had insisted on tracking Berg down at her friend's house and calling her immediately, asking what Berg, the acting head of the NCI's lung cancer research group, planned to do in response to this remarkable development.

"There had been the article in *The Times* and he was really excited about it and decided that since [lung cancer] was the leading cause of cancer death, NCI should at least be thinking about investigating it," Berg recalled of their conversation.

The new technology was not completely new to Berg. She had learned of the research on LDCT screening more than a year earlier during a visit from an epidemiologist at the University of Toronto, Anthony Miller, and understood its potential.

"I had just started at NCI when this guy Tony Miller came into my office and said he'd just been at a meeting in Varese, Italy," where Henschke and colleagues presented some preliminary results about their lung cancer screening program, and that "it looked promising and the NCI should look into it," she said.

Henschke had initiated her pioneering research program, the Early Lung Cancer Action Program, or ELCAP, as an effort to determine whether LDCT screening could help doctors identify lung cancers in their earliest stages. Launched in 1992 with another Weill Cornell radiologist, David Yankelevitz, the ELCAP project had by the time of the meeting in Italy screened about 1,000 patients. They had identified twenty-seven cancerous growths in those patients, all but one of which was resectable, meaning it could be removed surgically and potentially cured.[3] Given the nearly unstoppable threat posed by more advanced lung cancers, with a five-year survival rate below 20 percent, these were striking findings.

Those results offered a dose of optimism in a field where there had been little for decades. Following publication of *The Lancet* study, Henschke and Yankelevitz received hundreds of phone calls everyday from people interested in LDTC. By 2000, they had expanded ELCAP from two sites to more than ten.

A century ago, lung cancer was relatively rare, with death rates in the U.S. fewer than five per 100,000 people.[4] Ninety years later, rates were up twelve-fold.[5] In 2020, lung cancer killed an estimated 130,000 people in the U.S.,[6]

The demonstration of the promise of LDCT screening thus represented a watershed development, a potential turning point. But, as we will explain, intense resistance by some in the medical field, prolonged delays, and, again, the barriers to implementation meant that the benefits of this technology have been all too slow in reaching those who need it most.

Given the toll of this disease, there had been previous efforts to develop early-detection tests, to find tumors before the patients exhibited symptoms, but all had failed. There had been, for example, an attempt to detect lung cancer in asymptomatic patients in 1960 with the Northwest London Mass Radiography Service. It screened 55,000 men over the course of three years to determine if chest x-rays and sputum cytology could spot malignancies before they had grown or spread. But the study found no statistically significant improvements in survival rates between screened and unscreened groups.[7]

Numerous similar trials were launched over the next four decades, but none demonstrated any mortality benefits from screening.

The NCI started three large trials in the 1970s, one led by the Memorial Sloan-Kettering Cancer Center,[8] one led by Johns Hopkins University,[9] and one led by the Mayo Clinic.[10] The Sloan-Kettering and Johns Hopkins trials screened a combined 20,427 men who were given either annual chest x-rays or chest x-rays combined with sputum cytology (in which clinicians use microscopes to look for cancer cells in individuals' sputum). Again, there was disappointment. Following the subjects for five years, they found no difference in mortality rates between the screened and the unscreened groups.

The Mayo Clinic study looked at 9,211 male smokers, screening roughly half either with chest x-rays or chest x-rays and sputum cytology every four months. The other half, which was considered the control group, received x-rays or x-rays and sputum cytology as well, but only annually. In this case, the more intensely screened group actually showed a slightly higher lung cancer mortality after six years, though it was not statistically significant. This group had a mortality rate of 3.2 deaths per 1,000 person-years, while the control group, which received the annual screening, registered 3 deaths per 1,000 person-years.

A Czechoslovakian study published in 1986 similarly failed to demonstrate a benefit to the screening methods used at that time.[11] That study looked at 6,364 male smokers, comparing the results for those who received chest x-rays and sputum cytology twice a year with those who received no screening. The data showed that, after three years of testing, more cancers were detected in the screened group, but there was no difference between the two groups in the most important figure: cancer mortality.

The NCI conducted an even more comprehensive and ambitious x-ray–based trial from 1993 to 2001, the Prostate, Lung, Colorectal, and Ovarian Cancer Screening Trial. For the lung testing, it enrolled 154,901 men and women between 55 and 74 years of age, half of whom were screened annually with chest x-rays and half of whom received no screening. After thirteen years of follow-up, the study again found no significant difference in lung cancer mortality rates between the two groups and no significant difference in the stage of the detected cancers or their characteristics. The researchers concluded, disappointingly, that "annual screening with chest radiograph did not reduce lung cancer mortality compared with usual care."[12]

But while those older tests were proving fruitless, another technology was emerging: LDCT. The basic concepts underlying CT were introduced in the 1960s, and the first commercial CT scanners were developed in the early 1970s by researchers at the British conglomerate EMI (a project that was, according to some histories of the device, funded by profits from the sale of Beatles albums at EMI's music division).[13]

A CT scan essentially takes a series of x-rays, each creating images at different depths inside a patient's body, then assembles those images using computers to produce a highly detailed three-dimensional image, as though peering deep inside the patient's tissue.

Early CT scanners were poorly suited to lung screening. "They were revolutionary at the time, but compared to our current technology, they were slow and clunky," said Berg of the NCI. She recalled that when she did an oncology fellowship at the NCI in the early 1980s, scanning a patient's lungs took about one and a half hours. Today, a CT scan is done in seconds.

The individual images that make up a CT scan have also gotten more precise, meaning each image represents a detailed look inside a narrower segment of tissue. This has improved the technique's resolution and allowed radiologists to identify lung nodules—potentially cancerous growths—as tiny as several millimeters in diameter. That is far smaller than the abnormalities that traditional x-rays can consistently discern.

THE BREAKTHROUGH TECHNOLOGY ARRIVES, MAYBE

Imagine, by way of illustration, slicing through a watermelon and looking for seeds. If you cut thick wedges, seeds buried in the middle will remain hidden. Make your slices thin enough, though, and you'll see all of them. These narrow CT "slices" are key, because the success of lung cancer early detection—like cancer early detection generally—hinges on finding tumors when they are still small, harder to spot, and have yet to spread.

The first large-scale study of lung screening using the LDCT technology was published in 1996 by researchers at Japan's National Cancer Center Hospital.[14] They screened 1,369 patients at high risk for lung cancer twice a year from 1993 to 1995. The tests detected fifteen malignancies; of those, eleven were not picked up by traditional chest x-rays. That appeared to show the superiority of the LDCT scanners. Even more significant, fourteen of the fifteen cases were at stage I. At that stage this normally deadly cancer has cure rates as high as 80 percent to 90 percent.

In 1998, researchers at Japan's Shinshu University School of Medicine published a second, larger study.[15] It employed a mobile screening unit and tested 5,483 individuals selected from the general population, ages 40 to 74. The researchers found nineteen cases of lung cancer, only four of which could be discerned with chest x-rays, and 84 percent of which were at stage I.

"That was really the underpinning" of LDCT lung screening, Berg said. "The technology matured and that made it a feasible idea."

In the spring of 1999, several months before Klausner's phone call, Berg had already started exploring the possibility of launching a clinical trial in the U.S. to update the studies on the effectiveness of LDCT screening. That fall, just after the study's release, the NCI convened doctors and cancer scientists to discuss the project. In January 2000, Berg and her team proposed a large-scale, 50,000-person trial.

The cost: $250 million.

The NCI approved the plan. Known as the National Lung Screening Trial (NLST), this assault on the deadliest type of cancer was the most expensive such trial ever. It was launched in 2002 at thirty-three medical centers across the U.S.

Trials of cancer screening technologies are highly complex as well as, obviously, expensive, and, after weighing all the factors, experts often differ in their opinions not just on how they should be pursued, but even if they should be pursued at all. So it was not totally unexpected that some researchers argued against the massive NLST trial. But what was surprising was that two of the more outspoken opponents were Claudia Henschke and David Yankelevitz, among the test's greatest champions. Here was a chance to demonstrate, on perhaps the grandest scale possible, the effectiveness of the procedure they had spent nearly a decade investigating and promoting, yet they resisted the trial.

The two had consistently battled skeptics of the technology, and their careers were tightly associated with its development. But now their greatest concern over the proposed yearslong trial boiled down to a simple question—why wait? They argued that the earlier trials had proven the new technology a highly effective lifesaver. The evidence, they asserted, was powerful and beyond question. An enormous, enormously time-consuming trial to demonstrate that further would only delay a much wider rollout of the method as the medical profession waited for the results. It wasn't needed, they believed.

WAS THE WAIT WORTH IT?

Claudia Henschke had taken an indirect route to her career in medicine, but she brought with her a firm understanding of statistics and data analysis. Though her father was a well-known radiation oncologist, Ulrich Henschke, and her mother, Gisela Henschke, was also an oncologist, Claudia Henschke had first studied and earned a doctorate in mathematical statistics and computer science at the University of Georgia.

When she and her husband moved to Washington, D.C., after his appointment to a position at the NCI, Henschke took a position in the biostatistics department at Georgetown Medical School. But she soon changed course and decided that what she really wanted to do was work in medicine. She began her studies at the Howard University Medical School in 1974 and followed up with a residency in radiology at Brigham and Women's Hospital-Harvard Medical School. In 1983, she moved to Cornell University Medical College (now Weill Cornell Medicine) where she met Yankelevitz, who would become a research partner. The two, along with collaborators at other institutions, had launched the Early Lung Cancer Action Program in 1992 to determine if the promising new LDCT technology would be effective in early detection of lung cancer.

Given the positive results, Henschke, Yankelevitz, and their collaborators believed postponing the implementation of LDCT screening to wait on a decade-long trial was overly cautious. Thousands of patients who might have been cured would potentially die from advanced lung cancers that might have been caught through the new screening protocol. However, supporters of the NLST trial were convinced that moving forward in the absence of more comprehensive data was reckless. Some even raised questions about the design of the earlier, positive study that had been conducted by Henschke and Yankelevitz.

Peter Bach, director at that time of Memorial Sloan-Kettering's Center for Health Policy and Outcomes, was one of Henschke and Yankelevitz's antagonists. He argued that the issue was not nearly as straightforward as the researchers believed. "The evaluation of cancer screening approaches is complex, and involves many subtle epidemiologic concepts that can seem counterintuitive," he said in a critique.[16]

He was right in arguing that these evaluations can be difficult and less than straightforward; teasing out the actual mortality benefits of a screening method isn't necessarily as simple as demonstrating a shift to a higher percentage of earlier diagnoses. But subsequent events have shown that Bach's skepticism about this vital test was misplaced.

One issue cancer screening faces is the possibility of what is called lead-time bias. That's the idea that early detection of a cancer might not actually extend a person's life; it might just extend the time they live knowing they have cancer.

For instance, imagine a 65-year-old patient who undergoes a CT scan that detects a stage I lung cancer, when the patient has no symptoms. Suppose that cancer ultimately grows and causes his death ten years later. Now imagine, on the other hand, a patient with the same malignancy at the same age but who never gets screened. The growing lung cancer is discovered only after he develops symptoms, a persistent cough, at 73 years old. He also dies at age 75.

If you just looked at the first example and the time that had passed between the screening and death, and compared that with the second example, with the later diagnosis, it might appear that the screening had extended the life of the first person. He lived for ten years after the diagnosis, while the other person survived just two years after the diagnosis. In truth, in this example the patients die of lung cancer at 75 with or without the scan. That's lead-time bias and it does happen in the real world.

Overdiagnosis is another potential problem with some cancers, particularly those that are slow-growing and thus not life-threatening. Take the example of that 65-year-old patient again. At times, lung screening can detect what turn out to be indolent stage I tumors. But it is not always clear when such cancers are likely to be deadly. Aggressive treatments, such as risky surgeries or drug therapies, can inflict harm and, in some cases, actually kill the patient.

The solution medical science has devised to try to prevent such outcomes is the randomized controlled trial, or RCT. In this process, the people in the study are randomly assigned to one of two groups—an experimental group, which receives the intervention being evaluated, and a control arm, which does not get the treatment or test. By assigning people to those groups at random and treating them exactly the same, other than the intervention being evaluated, researchers assume that any differences in outcomes are due to that intervention and the intervention alone.

The first RCT to be detailed in the medical literature—an investigation of streptomycin for treating tuberculosis—was published in the *British Medical Journal* in 1948. Since then, RCTs have become the gold standard for testing effectiveness in medicine. Datasets from thousands of these trials are published every year. The NLST was to be a large RCT.

Henschke, Yankelevitz, and their allies felt strongly that the evidence was in and that there was too much at stake to withhold the test from people most at risk from the disease: smokers or former smokers. One of these allies, an epidemiologist, Olli Miettinen, wrote a commentary in *Cancer*, in 2000, titled "Screening for Lung Cancer: Do We Need Randomized Trials?"[17] At one medical conference, Henschke, Yankelevitz, and Miettinen battled with Berg of the NCI during an hourlong panel discussion about the need for a trial.

There was another reason behind the opposition to the long trial. Henschke and Yankelevitz were concerned that in subtle ways the trial's design disadvantaged LDCT and would, therefore, show that the technology was ineffective, or at least less effective than they had found it to be. If it failed in the trial, they feared, the costs of starting over would be so prohibitive that there would be no second chance.

If the NLST showed little or no benefit from LDCT lung screening, they worried, it might kill the idea forever. That was an unacceptable prospect, in their view.

But the adoption of important new medical techniques is never just a matter of producing favorable research data. There must be broad buy-in from regulatory agencies, professional bodies, insurers, specialists, and primary care physicians, an arduous process. A convincing trial is often an irreplaceable type of persuasion in developing a supportive consensus among the different stakeholders. With that in mind, the NLST went forward.

The long-awaited findings were released in November 2010, and the following summer the results were summarized in *The New England Journal of Medicine.* The trial found that screening people at high risk of lung cancer using the LDCT could lower mortality rates from the worst cancer killer in the country by as much as 20 percent.[18]

That was not the clear victory that anxious LDCT advocates had hoped for. Reducing by 20 percent the number of deaths from a disease that killed 130,000 people a year suggested that, to some degree, the trial was a success. But Henschke and Yankelevitz were disappointed that the results fell so far short of what they were convinced was the technique's true benefit, a 60 percent to 80 percent reduction, and they laid out the reasons they felt the trial's design minimized the success rate.

For starters, the trial used what is called a stop-screen design. The subjects were given three screenings over two years; then the screenings were halted. They were then monitored for an average of 6.5 additional years without more screening. The advantage of the stop-screen design is lower costs—screening is typically the most expensive part of a trial, and reducing the number of screening rounds prevents costs from climbing even higher.

But stopping the screening so early can dilute the overall results, some experts argue. Lung cancers that arose and killed patients during that 6.5-year follow-up period counted as participant deaths even though no screening had taken place during those later years. In fact, roughly one-third of the lung cancer diagnoses made in the trial's screening group came after screening had ended. Might continued screening have picked up those cancers at an early stage, allowing them to be treated successfully? That question went unanswered.

Also, a percentage of lung tumors are potentially lethal but slow in developing. In the group that underwent screenings, those cancers most likely would have been found and surgically removed at some point. In the control group, with no screenings, those cancers likely went undetected. Yet if they caused the death of the subjects after the trial ended, they were not counted in the final results. This, too, may have diminished the relative benefits of screening.

Another issue that raised questions about the validity of the data was that each of the thirty-three facilities participating in the trial could handle the treatment of any nodules detected by LDCT—suspected cancers—as they wished. Without a standard protocol for those treatments, there was no uniformity in the outcomes.

As Paul Pinsky, one of the NCI investigators on the trial, testified during a hearing on the LDCT screening, "diagnostic follow-up, as well as treatment, was conducted outside of the auspices of the NLST."[19] Careful treatment thus could have produced cures of the early-stage cancers, while weaker treatment might have resulted in deaths, with no means of distinguishing between them in the study results.

Another important question was raised about the study results based on the overall design. The NLST did not find that LDCT screening cuts lung cancer mortality by 20 percent in some type of overall fixed sense that could be expected under all circumstances in the future. Instead, it found that only under the specific conditions established for that specific trial (the three rounds of screening, the six years of follow-up, the nonstandardized follow-up procedures and treatment of nodules), LDCT screening yielded that result. And, importantly, this was exactly the result the researchers had targeted in advance—the benchmark for effectiveness they had hoped to hit.

Clinical trials are expensive, and while the NLST was better funded than most, its resources were still limited. So the trial's planners had considered the resources available to them and attempted to predict what, just with the amount of screening they did have funding to complete, the mortality benefit of an effective LDCT program would show. Under those narrow conditions, the figure they arrived at was 20 percent—meaning that if the NLST showed that lung screening cut cancer deaths by 20 percent, LDCT testing could be considered a success.

Given that built-in limitation and their pretrial expectations, the researchers did something significant—when, eight years in, the screening had produced the 20 percent benefit, the trial was stopped two years early. It had hit its target. It had proved, in their eyes, that lung screening worked, even if the figure fell short of what LDCT supporters had experienced in trials without such limits.

Henschke and Yankelevitz were not alone in observing the limitations of the NLST. NCI's Berg also has suggested that had participants been subject to more rounds of screening, the demonstrated benefit would have been much higher. She has cited data suggesting that the five-year survival rate observed in the study was actually between 50 percent and 55 percent.[20]

In the *New England Journal of Medicine* article sharing the NLST results, the trial's researchers themselves acknowledged that the decline in the rate of death "may be larger than the 20 percent reduction observed with only three rounds of screening."

Brady McKee, a radiologist who ran lung cancer screening at Lahey Hospital and Medical Center in Burlington, Massachusetts, which has one of the largest screening programs in the country, said he believed that the true mortality reduction is "enormously higher" than 20 percent.

Even so, the sides remained entrenched in their positions and the debate continued for a number of years following the trial—which should be regarded as a reflection of the way personalities, and not just data, can influence how the medical profession assesses and uses early-detection screening.

Bach, of Memorial Sloan-Kettering, wrote in *Slate* in 2010 that the NLST study "showed that regular scans prevented one in five lung cancer deaths, which means that four out of five sneaked through."[21]

". . . screening is not a panacea," he went on. "Not even close."

In an interview with *The New York Times* several years ago, Eric Topol, chair of innovative medicine at Scripps Research and the former chair of cardiology at the Cleveland Clinic, said the effectiveness of lung cancer screening was "so bad that it's hard to make it worse." To support this assertion he cited, among other things, the technique's supposedly high false positive rate.[22]

Some experts challenged his comment online, and Topol responded by referencing an academic study that, he claimed, supported his assessment. But one author of that study showed up in Topol's Twitter feed and insisted that, in fact, lung screening was far more effective than he had represented.[23]

Another expert who asserted that the benefits were modest was Otis Brawley, the chief medical and scientific officer at the American Cancer Society. He wrote in an editorial in *The Cancer Letter* in 2014: "Low dose CT when done well has the potential of reducing relative risk of lung cancer death by about 20 percent."[24]

While a 20 percent mortality reduction is substantial, meaning thousands of people a year would not die earlier from the disease than might be ordinarily expected, the deeper problem, which supporters had warned about, is that it wasn't so overwhelming as to persuade LDCT's skeptics that a full-scale, heavily funded, well-publicized rollout was justified. Such a rollout ought to have included funding for a large-scale advertising campaign using mass media and social media. While Henschke and Yankelevitz had feared that the NLST results and the ensuing debate might kill off this early-detection protocol, instead, it produced a sort of paralysis, draining the energy from the movements for action. The unfortunate result: nearly a decade after the massive trial ended, only about 4.5 percent of those at high risk of lung cancer are being screened with LDCT.

"It took twenty years to embark on a real research program that could prove that lung cancer screening works," said Raja Flores, chief of thoracic surgery at Mount Sinai Health Systems in New York and a sometime collaborator with Henschke and Yankelevitz. "So finally they did it. Finally [LDCT] is proven to work. And now they're minimizing its effects."

BALANCING THE RISKS OF OVERTREATMENT AND UNDERTREATMENT

Two common but important concerns with any screening protocol are false negatives—when the test says you don't have a disease but, in fact, you do—and false positives—when the test says you do have the disease, but you do not. For most tests, there is a natural tension between the two. The more steps taken to sharpen the assessments and reduce false negatives, the greater the likelihood that the extra scrutiny may increase false positives, and vice versa.

In lung screening, when radiologists read a patient's LDCT scan they search for abnormal features—spots, nodules, or lesions—that are not typically present in healthy lungs. The challenge is, while these features can indicate the presence of cancer, they can also be caused by other noncancerous factors, including infections, scarring, or inflammation. In practice, it can be difficult to distinguish between the two, even for highly skilled physicians.

That is why doctors and early-detection specialists take what are often complex precautions to try to strike a reasonable balance between the extremes of undertreatment and overtreatment that can result from inaccurate test results, realizing that neither can be eliminated entirely. But the concern over false positives and the potential for subjecting patients to unnecessary invasive treatments is a fear that critics of LDCT testing have used to raise further doubts about its efficacy.

The data clearly shows, however, that the problem of unnecessary, invasive follow-up procedures for false positives detected by LDCT is manageable. In the NLST, the overwhelming majority of follow-up procedures were, in fact, noninvasive. For instance, in 50 percent of cases, the follow-up for a detected nodule consisted of another CT scan. In 14 percent of the cases it involved an x-ray, while in 8.3 percent the follow-up involved another type of sophisticated test, PET imaging. That stands for positron emission tomography, in which a radioactive tracer drug is injected into the patient, where it helps reveal normal and abnormal metabolic activity of the cells in tissue and organs.

Biopsies were done in just 1.8 percent of the cases, while a bronchoscopy, in which a thin imaging wire, a bronchoscope, is inserted in the nose or mouth, allowing the doctor to see into the lungs and collect cells for testing, was done in 3.8 percent of the cases. A surgical procedure was conducted in 4 percent of the cases. Importantly, those percentages are for both the false positive and true positive findings from the LDCT screening. Just 0.07 percent—seven one-hundredths of 1 percent—of the unnecessary follow-up from false positives resulted in a major complication.

Skeptics highlighted that 245 patients in the trial experienced complications from follow-up procedures. But of those, 184 had lung cancer, had correctly tested positive, and needed some type of treatment.

Today, false positive rates for initial scans run between 10 percent and 14 percent. But that rate declines further, to 6 percent, when the radiologist is able to compare a patient's imaging to previous tests.[25]

THE USES, AND ABUSES, OF EVIDENCE-BASED MEDICINE

Certainly, some legitimate concerns have been raised about established screening practices based on the evidence supplied through trials.

Part of this story begins in the early 1950s with Tom Chalmers, a civilian physician working with the U.S. Army in Kyoto, Japan, who was overseeing the treatment of Korean War soldiers with hepatitis. At that time, the standard treatment for hepatitis was long periods of bed rest. If the soldiers were allowed to move freely before overcoming the illness, it was believed, they risked permanent damage to their health. For Chalmers and his staff, this meant a constant headache as they tried to keep a ward filled with bored young men confined to their beds.

Chalmers found when he looked into the question that the evidence behind the resting treatment was incomplete at best. To learn for themselves, Chalmers and his colleagues set up a trial, randomly assigning 250 hepatitis patients to one of two groups—one in which soldiers were treated with bed rest, and a second in which they were allowed to move around about as much as they wanted.

When the data was tabulated, Chalmers found that not only was bed rest not essential, it actually lengthened the duration of the recoveries. And examining the patients a year later, Chalmers found no long-term differences between the two groups. Chalmers's trial evidence provided strong support for possible changes in treatment of a serious illness.

The researchers published a paper in 1955 detailing the findings. Four years later, a University of Illinois medical student named David Sackett came across the study when he was trying to decide how best to treat a teenage hepatitis patient. Bed rest was still the prescribed course of treatment for the condition but, armed with Chalmers' study, Sackett decided to let his patient move about as much as he liked.

"He did, and his clinical course was uneventful," Sackett recalled.[26]

For Sackett, the experience taught him that "accepted" medical practices, frequently unquestioned or tested, too often were embraced through habit and unthinking adherence to past practices. This insight animated the rest of Sackett's career and helped change the course of medical research and practice.

Over the next fifty years, Sackett and a handful of like-minded clinicians, including a Scottish doctor, Archibald Cochrane, and a Yale School of Medicine professor, Alvan Feinstein, as well as Chalmers, promoted the use of carefully organized clinical studies and reviews of the scientific literature to provide the best outcomes for patients.

In the 1960s, Sackett founded Canada's first department of clinical epidemiology at McMaster University, which employed such studies. In 1991 a former student of his, Gordon Guyatt, published a one-page editorial in the medical journal ACP Journal Club, that gave this critical scientific practice its name.[27] Guyatt called it "evidence-based medicine," or EBM.

PREVENTIVE MEDICINE GETS A FEDERAL OVERSEER, AND MORE QUESTIONS

A key player in applying EBM to cancer early detection is the U.S. Preventive Services Task Force. It is an expert panel within the federal Department of Health and Human Services that evaluates the effectiveness of screening and other tools used in preventive medicine, applying rigorous analysis of testing and trial data.

Should children younger than 5 get fluoride supplements to strengthen their teeth? The task force has looked into the research and has a recommendation (yes, they should). Should men aged 65 or above get ultrasounds to check for abdominal aortic aneurysm? Chances are their doctors will decide based on guidelines from the task force (yes, in many circumstances they should).

Formed in 1984, the organization has become one of the most influential bodies in medicine, a major player in guiding physician practices as well as health insurance coverage decisions. Its influence grew even further after the 2010 passage of the Affordable Care Act, which mandated insurance companies to cover preventive services recommended by the Preventive Services Task Force. (In March 2023, the Federal Dis-

trict Court for the Northern District of Texas overturned this portion
of the law. As of June 2023, the court ruling had been stayed and the
government is expected to appeal, but if the court's decision ultimately
stands, insurers will no longer be required to cover these recommended services, including several kinds of cancer screening.)

Steven Woolf, a professor of family medicine and population
health at Virginia Commonwealth University, joined the task force in
1987, when it was still in its formative years, and became one of its first
staff science advisers. When he joined, the organization was working
to develop a standard placard that doctors could keep in their offices
summarizing the preventive services people should receive at different ages. It was based on a similar chart produced by the Canadian
Task Force on Preventive Health Care, an organization that helped
inspire the creation of the U.S. task force. (An original member of the
Canadian task force, founded a decade before the U.S. version, was
David Sackett of McMaster University.)

"It was sort of a colorful fold-out that showed, you know, for ages
18 to 24, these are the [preventive services] you should get, and if
you're 25 to 49, this is what you should get, and so on," Woolf said.
"And I thought, this is fabulous. This is what I want to do."

By the time he joined the task force full time, the simple chart had
become a series of two-page documents, each detailing the case for a
particular test or screening. The list included things like cholesterol
testing and screening for depression. Cancer screening also figured
prominently in the task force's charts.

The result of this effort to improve healthcare outcomes began as
a simple placard and then became a series of two-pagers and ultimately morphed into a 400-page book published by the task force in 1989.

Even with this sort of intensive analysis, making the right call on early-detection tests can be difficult, Woolf acknowledged. He cited his own
experience evaluating colon cancer screening methods during his early
years with the task force. At that time, the mid-1980s, the task force did

not recommend colonoscopies due to what it said was a lack of evidence showing that the procedure actually reduced deaths from colon cancer.

"The specialists at the National Cancer Institute and the American Cancer Society were furious with us because they were in the middle of trying to promote this and they [were] also watching how many people [were] dying from the disease," Woolf said. "And I was in the position as this young person saying in a very nerdy way, 'I'm sorry, it doesn't meet our evidence standards.'"

A few years later, further studies supported the use of colonoscopies as a tool for detecting colon cancers. "By the early nineties we were saying, 'Oh yeah, you should get screened for colon cancer,'" Woolf said. "And, you know, the guilt that weighed on me for many years is how many people died from colon cancer due to not getting screened when it turns out it was effective."

Woolf's experience with colonoscopy shows how difficult making these calls can be, particularly in the early days of a technology, when the data from trials or implementation may be limited. It also suggests why, despite the evidence supporting LDCT, lung screening has proved so contentious. After all, while Henschke and Yankelevitz's work was not, perhaps, conclusive to some doctors, it unquestionably showed substantial promise.

MEDICARE'S FLIP-FLOP ON LUNG TESTING

In 2014, the question of early detection of lung cancer came before the Medicare Evidence Development & Coverage Advisory Committee, where a group of researchers and clinicians were tasked with recommending whether Medicare, the large federal healthcare program for people over 65, should cover LDCT screening. During the research process, Memorial Sloan-Kettering's Peter Bach summed up the dispute as being about "basic questions of extrapolation."

"Was this group study generalizable?" he asked. "Are the findings [from the NLST] in terms of mortality, false positives, and adherence generalizable? Were the settings generalizable?"

Bach concluded that he was satisfied the results were, in fact, generalizable and that the panel could expect LDCT screening to reduce lung cancer deaths when put into wide practice, if not to the degree promised by Henschke and Yankelevitz.[28]

Woolf, who had since left the U.S. Preventive Services Task Force, served as an expert on the Medicare committee, and he argued that patients in a study might act differently than people outside it. Outside the context of a clinical study, patients were less likely to adhere to recommended screenings and follow-up, he said, and that the quality of evaluation and treatment protocols were thus likely to vary considerably across hospitals and patient populations.[29]

When it was time to decide, the Medicare Evidence Development & Coverage Advisory Committee voted to reject coverage for LDCT lung cancer screening.

"I thought there would be a tsunami of screening and that it would be somewhat indiscriminate, that it wouldn't be done thoughtfully," said Michael Gould, another panelist and a health services researcher at Kaiser Permanente Southern California. "Were we ready for it? Did we have the capacity? Was it going to be complete chaos in radiology departments and pulmonary practices following up on all the abnormal findings?"

The reality? In places where LDCT was implemented, none of these things came to pass. Gould, it turned out, changed his mind and his conclusion.

"If I had ambivalence before about screening, and I did," Gould said, "I think it has now become indefensible not to offer screening."

The results have been positive. Real-world screening programs have significantly reduced the number of late-stage lung cancer patients in their communities, and additional high-quality studies have reinforced the positive results of the NLST trial.

This includes another large-scale trial, the Nederlands–Leuvens Longkanker Screenings Onderzoek (NELSON) trial, a 15,000-subject Dutch-Belgian study launched in 2003. Half the subjects were screened four times over five and a half years and followed for at least another ten years, through 2015.[30] The findings were even more positive than the big U.S. trial, demonstrating a 26 percent reduction in lung cancer mortality in men and a 61 percent reduction in women.

More recently, Henschke and Yankelevitz published new ELCAP data providing further evidence that screening can boost twenty-year lung cancer survival rates to over 80 percent.[31]

The tide in the long battle was turning.

In 2013, the U.S. Preventive Services Task Force recommended that individuals at high risk for lung cancer undergo annual LDCT screening. In addition to providing a powerful endorsement of the procedure to doctors, the task force recommendation meant that private insurers were obligated to cover the screening free of charge.

In 2015, Medicare rejected the earlier negative Medicare Evidence Development & Coverage Advisory Committee recommendations and added LDCT screening to its coverage.

Since then, support for lung screening has grown even stronger. In 2021, the U.S. Preventive Services Task Force updated its guidelines. It expanded the group of individuals recommended for screening from the original cohort—adults aged 55 to 80 with a thirty-pack-year smoking history, who had smoked within the last fifteen years—to adults aged 50 to 80 with a twenty-pack-year smoking history who had smoked within the last fifteen years. (A "pack-year" is the numbers of cigarette packs smoked per day multiplied by the number of years the patient smoked.)[32]

Even with that broadening of the eligibility requirements, a study found that only about 65 percent of people diagnosed with lung cancer would be eligible for LDCT screening, an indication that it may need to take further steps to loosen eligibility and potentially save more lives.[33]

The National Comprehensive Cancer Network, a collection of the leading cancer treatment centers in the U.S., recommends screening fifty- to eighty-year-olds with a twenty-pack-year smoking history regardless of how recently they have smoked, provided they have an additional risk factor like a family history of the disease or exposure to certain lung carcinogens.[34]

Even those endorsements have not had the needed impact. Early detection of lung cancer has languished. In the U.S., still only about 4.5 percent of the eligible population is being screened. Outside the U.S. the number is even lower. There is not nearly enough communication and advertising to persuade the people at risk to get screened regularly.

This remains true even as the tests improve. Newer generations of the LDCT devices emit less radiation, thus reducing the risk of health problems due to the exposure. And computer algorithms have been developed that could help identify nodules and other abnormalities in the images much faster and, in some cases, more effectively than radiologists, reducing the number of false readings.

"These computer-aided methods could potentially allow even earlier diagnosis, reduce diagnostic evaluations and anxiety for benign nodules, and increase consistency and confidence in lesion management," five researchers concluded in a 2020 report on LDCT technology in the periodical *Radiology: Imaging Cancer.*[35]

Other factors appear to be at work in the disappointing reality of the low uptake of the screening—and we provide a telling example in a later chapter on what appear to be some of the societal challenges to improved use of this lifesaving tool. One clear factor seems to be that lung cancer overwhelmingly affects smokers, a group that is disproportionately made up of lower-income people who are badly underserved by the healthcare system. And because of the link to smoking, lung cancer has a social stigma not attached to most other cancers. It is believed that these factors have discouraged some smokers from seeking screening and made lung cancer a less sympathetic target for philanthropic and government support. That has limited the funds available to advertise and drive acceptance of LDCT screening, even though 130,000 lives a year are at stake.

To turn around this disappointing reality, the government and medical community ought to pursue a number of initiatives: the Centers for Disease Control and Prevention, as well as other government health policy agencies, should launch a large-scale public information campaign on the benefits of and need for lung cancer screening among those at risk, at least on a scale of its ongoing efforts, over a period of years, to make people aware of the benefits of colonoscopies; more government funding must be allocated to better training of primary physicians and radiologists on LDCT screening; and appropriate community organizations as well as healthcare nonprofits and philanthropies should be invited to partner with medical providers and government agencies to spread awareness of LDCT screening and its benefits.

There are 130,000 reasons why it is worth the effort.

CHAPTER 4

HOW TO FIX A GOOD TEST GONE BAD:

CLEANING UP THE MESS IN PROSTATE AND BREAST CANCER SCREENING

WE HAVE DESCRIBED SOME OF THE SETBACKS AND CHALLENGES early-detection tests have faced, even when the science seems overwhelmingly positive. But there is an important reason for the frustrating fits and starts—the medical system's adherence to an ancient Latin medical principle: Primum non nocere. First, do no harm.

Few if any industries require so much care, oversight, rigor, expense, and repetition in the testing of new products and procedures before consumers are allowed to access them as medicine. And there is good reason for that. The medical system has been racked on occasion by the scandalous harm caused by treatments that inflicted terrible pain and devastating consequences on patients, no matter how well-meaning. Doctors know that they operate on an ethical foundation that insists that first, do no harm. That has been and will continue to be a critical hurdle that early-detection tests must overcome before wide application, protecting the safety of patients.

What makes that particularly challenging is the reality that early-detection screening typically focuses on patients who exhibit no symptoms, who are likely to appear healthy. Any follow-up tests or treatments for those found to have abnormalities, or suspected abnormalities, can be painful and risky. No test is perfect, and thus false positives and some instances of overtreatment are inevitable. How many such instances are too many compared with the lives saved? A medical establishment that counts "first, do no harm" as a guiding maxim feels uneasy, understandably, about the potential for needless treatments.

Complicating the process further is the fact that testing is driven in large part by statistical conventions like probability, likelihood, estimates. Randomized controlled trials try to reduce the margins for error, sharpen those probabilities, develop reliable models, and add weight to decisions about medical testing. Screening is an art of approximation, using limited data to draw wider conclusions that are reasonable and, most likely, accurate. But there are limits and there is frequently debate about where boundaries should be set.

There is a short story by the great Argentinian writer Jorge Luis Borges called "On Rigor in Science" that draws out this truth with an amusing but revealing parable. The story, published in 1946, is one paragraph long. It is written as though it was an excerpt from a seventeenth-century description of an empire where cartographers grew so zealous in making maps of ever-greater precision that they ultimately made one that was the size of the empire itself, an exact, full-sized replica. That, of course, rendered the map both perfect and useless.

Clinical trials face a similar dilemma. At root, they simply rely on and build models, sophisticated models that use those statistical projections. Ideally, they are good models, with thoughtfully structured processes and protocols and carefully selected patient cohorts, all designed to predict as well as possible how a test, drug or procedure will perform when it enters clinical practice in the real world. A trial isn't the real world, though, and it never can be without running into the same problem faced by Borges's mapmakers. And this inevitable gap between the environment of a clinical trial and the real-world circumstances it aims to reflect means that there will always be potential for uncertainty, some risk, and a need to balance those risks against the potential rewards, saving many thousands of lives.

Those considerations are a useful place to begin to examine the mess that followed the introduction in 1994 of a screening test for prostate cancer, called prostate-specific antigen, or PSA. The test faced a number of challenges, including a relatively high false positive rate and the fact that, even among true positives, many of the cancers identified were slow-growing and did not necessarily require treatment. Nonetheless, PSA testing undeniably contributed to a significant decline in prostate cancer deaths, and, while the medical community was, perhaps, initially unprepared to deal with its complexities, physicians are becoming more sophisticated in their use of it, limiting its downsides while continuing to save lives.

A key lesson was that the screening method needed to be embedded in a more comprehensive analytical process with thoughtful checks against misreadings. The PSA test should be treated as just the first step in data collection. Any indications of malignant growths need to be followed up carefully with other types of testing and evaluation to separate genuine cancerous growths requiring medical interventions from either indolent growths or readings caused by factors unrelated to cancer. That is a lesson learned repeatedly by the medical profession, a lesson that has enhanced early-detection capabilities and the safety of patients.

THE PSA PROBLEM:
THE ANTIGEN IS PRESENT
FOR MANY REASONS

PSA, a protein produced by the prostate gland, plays an important role in reproduction, breaking down proteins in semen to enable sperm motility. It is normally present in the blood at low levels, and concerns about possible diseases rise as PSA levels rise.

Throughout the 1960s and 1970s, the protein was identified by several research groups working independently, making credit for its discovery unclear.[1] One of the first researchers to isolate the molecule was a Japanese scientist, Mitsuwo Hara, who identified it in the late 1960s (calling it γ-seminoprotein) as part of work investigating semen proteins that could be used as evidence in rape cases. Several years later, Richard Ablin, a pathologist at the University of Arizona College of Medicine, detected a pair of prostate proteins as part of studies into the immunological characteristics of prostate tissue. The first of those, prostatic acid phosphatase, was already well-known, having been identified some forty years prior. The second was a protein that Ablin and his colleagues labeled "prostate-specific antigen."

Meanwhile, Carl Beling and Tien Shun Li, fertility researchers at Cornell University Medical College, were studying semen proteins with the aim of developing new methods for treating male infertility. They also identified PSA, which they called the E1 antigen. And several years later, forensic scientist George Sensabaugh, following in Hara's footsteps, identified the same protein as a potential marker in rape investigations, calling it p30. Finally, in 1979, Ming Chu and Ming Wang, researchers at Roswell Park Memorial Institute, identified the protein in prostate tissue and called it PA, for "prostate antigen."

It took researchers thirteen years to establish that all of these molecules were, in fact, the same protein, PSA. By that time, tests for PSA levels were already being used to monitor prostate cancer patients for recurrence of the disease. A few years later, the test received FDA approval as a prostate cancer screening tool for the general population.

That is where the test ran into trouble.

From the beginning, it was clear that PSA was found not only in prostate gland tumors but also in healthy prostate tissue and prostate tissue affected by conditions like prostatitis (inflammation of the gland) and benign prostatic hyperplasia (an enlarged gland), common in older men. In other words, PSA, while "prostate-specific," wasn't "prostate-cancer-specific." (In fact, researchers later determined that PSA is not even strictly prostate-specific either.)

When scientists at Stanford University published, in 1987, one of the first clinical studies of PSA as a prostate cancer biomarker, they were quite clear on this limitation. They wrote that the elevation in PSA caused by benign hyperplasia "precludes the use of the PSA concentration as a means of screening for prostatic cancer."[2]

That determination underscored the dilemma raised by the PSA test. If doctors raised the threshold high enough to exclude benign prostate disease, they would miss so many cancer cases it would make the marker far less useful. On the other hand, if they lowered the screening level enough to detect the bulk of cancers early, they would run into a cascade of false positives caused by the presence of PSA from those other factors.

As doctors have come to appreciate, using PSA for population-wide screening doesn't just, at times, pull in healthy men for unnecessary follow-up, it also singles out many men who have slow-growing prostate cancers, tumors that would most likely never threaten their lives if left undetected. Some of those patients would then face the prospect of surgery for prostatectomies—and possible lifelong complications, such as impotence or incontinence—that they could have safely gone without. Such slow-growing cancers are, in fact, not uncommon. Autopsy studies have found that more than 30 percent of men over 70 have an undetected prostate cancer at the time of death.[3]

Given these limitations, how did PSA become one of the most widely used tools in cancer screening, with tens of millions of tests performed each year?

Money, of course, was a factor. In his 2014 book, *The Great Prostate Hoax: How Big Medicine Hijacked the PSA Test and Caused a Public Health Disaster*, Ablin recounts how the PSA test became the foundation of a multibillion-dollar-a-year business. At the peak, he writes, about 30 million PSA tests were administered every year. Around a million prostate biopsies were done as follow-ups, and about 100,000 prostatectomies were done to remove cancers found through this screening.

Every one of those tests and procedures (which do not include prostate cancer treatments like chemotherapy or radiation) generates income—for physicians, for labs, for diagnostics companies, and for hospital systems. Doctors may not have consciously ordered unnecessary PSA tests to drive profits, but Ablin quotes Otis Brawley, the former American Cancer Society chief medical and scientific officer, paraphrasing a famous Upton Sinclair quote, "If your income is dependent on you not understanding something, it is very easy not to understand something."[4]

But with the PSA test as well as other complex types of medical screening, the answers to these concerns are rarely black and white. In this case, the reason many doctors continued to order the PSA tests is the many instances in which they work, of course, helping to identify and stop dangerous malignancies—assuming that the approach is cautious and methodical with plenty of safeguards.

The test was initially approved in 1986 as a tool just for managing the care of men already diagnosed with prostate cancer. In 1994, the FDA approved it as a general screening test in combination with the commonly used digital rectal examination for men over 50, which led to greater use. Over the next twenty-five years, prostate cancer death rates in the U.S. were cut nearly in half, while the number of metastatic cases fell by more than 70 percent, exceptional outcomes.[5]

Throughout most of this period, the U.S. Preventive Services Task Force maintained a grade of "I" for PSA screening, indicating that it considered the evidence either for or against the test to be insufficient to make a recommendation. In 2008, concerns over overdiagnosis and overtreatment were growing and the task force changed its grade to a "D," for men over 75, meaning it recommended that men of this age not undergo PSA testing.[6] The task force was not through. In late 2011, it updated its guidelines again to expand this "D" rating to all age groups.

Death rates initially held steady following these updates, but the number of cases of late-stage, metastatic prostate cancer began rising in 2012. After this reversal, the task force again reviewed its guideline. In a turnaround, it revised the guideline in 2018 to maintain the "D" grade for men over 70 but gave a "C" rating for men ages 55 to 69, meaning they should consider PSA screening in consultation with their doctors.

EVALUATING CONTRADICTORY TRIAL FINDINGS

In the case of PSA screening, two large RCTs were conducted. There were the Prostate, Lung, Colorectal, and Ovarian (PLCO) Cancer

Screening Trial run by the NCI, which screened 76,683 U.S. men between the ages of 55 and 74, and the European Randomized Study of Screening for Prostate Cancer (ERSPC), which looked at 161,394 men between the ages of 55 and 69 in eight European countries. After testing and then thirteen years of follow-up, the ERSPC reported in 2014 that PSA testing reduced prostate cancer mortality in the screened group by 27 percent.[7] At fifteen years of follow-up, in 2017, the PLCO reported that PSA testing provided no mortality benefit.[8]

How could that be?

As we wrote in regard to the lung cancer screening RCT, trial results are highly dependent on the design. And the PLCO had a major design flaw. The study was set up as a typical RCT, with an intervention arm consisting of men who received PSA testing and a control arm of men who did not. After a number of years of testing and follow-up, the researchers then compared the prostate cancer mortality of men in the intervention group to those in the control group to see what, if any, differences could be observed in outcomes.

The problem was that the men in the intervention group were not the only ones receiving PSA testing. Almost all the men in the control arm, approximately 90 percent, also underwent PSA testing at some point during the trial. In fact, during the follow-up portion of the PLCO—years seven through thirteen—men in the control arm underwent more PSA testing than the men in the intervention arm. That, of course, runs counter to what should have happened in a well-designed and properly administered trial.

This phenomenon, when some members of the control arm receive the procedure being tested in the intervention arm, is called contamination. It's a challenge for many RCTs, and particularly for RCTs evaluating interventions that have become commonplace in clinical practice. The PLCO began enrolling patients in 1993 and ended enrollment in 2001. During that period, PSA testing exploded throughout the U.S., becoming, essentially, the standard of care for men in the age range enrolled in the trial. It's little surprise, therefore, that the PLCO found no difference in prostate cancer mortality between the intervention and control arms. With 90 percent contamination, there was effectively no control arm.

Estimates of contamination in the other large-scale trial, the ERSPC, were lower, but still a substantial 30 percent of the men in the trial's control group had taken the PSA test. That could not erase the differences between the two arms entirely, but may have reduced the prostate cancer mortality rate to the 27 percent level observed. With less contamination, the PLCO would very likely have shown a similar benefit.

In fact, when an international group of statisticians reanalyzed the PLCO data to try to account for the effects of the control group contamination, they calculated that PSA testing reduced prostate cancer deaths by about 25 percent to 30 percent. Publishing their findings in the Annals of Internal Medicine in 2017, they wrote that their analysis suggested that use of PSA screening "can significantly reduce the risk for prostate cancer death."[9]

All that evidence supports the conclusion that PSA testing, even if flawed, saves lives. The trials, the reanalysis of the PLCO, the epidemiological data showing a large decline in prostate cancer deaths following the advent of widespread PSA testing, and the increases in metastatic disease following a pullback in testing—it all reinforces a justified belief in the success of this early-detection tool.

The key question, then, is at what cost?

The positive results aside, prostate cancer screening remains complicated by the large number of cases of indolent disease that the PSA test detects. The ERSPC trial found that for every prostate cancer death prevented, doctors had identified another twenty-seven cancers that could have been safely left untreated. Many of these patients are treated, however. In 2010, almost half of the U.S. men diagnosed with low-risk prostate cancer received a radical prostatectomy—removal of the prostate and surrounding tissue—as their initial therapy.[10]

Again, the procedure can induce serious side effects, including impotence, incontinence, and the small but ever-present risks that accompany any major surgery. And yet the dangers of leaving prostate cancer untreated can be far worse. The five-year survival rate of localized prostate cancer, the stage at which the PSA test often detects it, is almost 100 percent. For more advanced metastatic disease, it's just over 30 percent.[11] That is a sobering contrast.

The PSA test is easy to administer. It can be ordered as one of the battery of routine blood tests men often get during their annual health checkups. On its face, this would seem a strength, but it has actually contributed to the problems.

Andrew Vickers is a biostatistician and research methodologist at Memorial Sloan-Kettering Cancer Center whose work focuses primarily on prostate cancer screening. A few years ago he coauthored an editorial in the journal *European Urology* with a title that neatly sums up the current PSA situation: "It Ain't What You Do, It's The Way You Do It . . ."[12] In his view, the PSA test is a potentially excellent screening tool but one that has been used carelessly for part of its history and that "the way you do it" needs to be improved.

"There's been a lot of misuse," he said. "And that's not unusual. You've got a sort of lack of knowledge. PSA tests are often done in primary care where, you know, doctors can't be experts on everything."

He added, "The problem with using PSA is you have to be specific. Once you have an elevated PSA you have to say, 'Okay, let's do a lot of other things to make sure this guy is really at high risk of a bad prostate cancer.'"

PSA is fairly sensitive as cancer markers go. If a prostate cancer is there, there is a good chance it will be detected. It's not, however, very specific, given that other noncancerous conditions can also lead to an elevated score.

For instance, among men with a score between 4 and 10 nano-grams per milliliter of blood—a level that would typically trigger a decision to do a biopsy—only about 25 percent will actually have pros-tate cancer.

Prostate cancers are graded according to what is known as the Gleason Score, named for pathologist Donald Gleason, who devel-oped the system in the 1960s. This scoring system focuses on what the cancer tissue actually looks like under a microscope and an as-sessment of how much it resembles normal tissue. In Gleason scor-ing, tissue in a tumor sample is graded 1 to 5, with 1 meaning it looks basically normal and 5 meaning it is severely malformed, or "dedif-ferentiated," and more likely dangerous.

A Gleason Score consists of two numbers that are added together—one representing the appearance of the most common score in the sample, the predominant tissue pattern visible, and the other repre-senting the second-most common pattern visible. For instance, a bi-opsy where tissue with a grade of 3 was the most common and tissue with a grade of 2 was the next-most common would receive a Gleason Score of 5. The higher the score, the more likely that the cancer will grow aggressively and threaten the life of the patient.

Gleason scores are typically further divided into grade groups, with a Gleason Score of 6 or lower falling into Grade Group 1, the lowest risk category. Grade Group 2 consists of patients with a 3+4 Gleason Score of 7, meaning grade 3 tissue is the most common in their biopsy and grade 4 tissue is the next-most common. Group 3 consists of patients with a 4+3 Gleason 7, meaning grade 4 tissue is the most common and grade 3 cells are the next-most common. Patients with a Gleason Score of 8 are considered Group 4, and patients with Gleason scores of 9 or 10 are Group 5.

A Gleason Score of 6 or below—Grade Group 1—is generally con-sidered low risk. And yet, Vickers noted, throughout the 1990s and early

2000s, "if you had a Gleason 6 cancer, almost all of those men were treated." Even worse, he added, many of them were treated poorly.

IN PROSTATE SURGERY, PROOF THAT EXPERIENCE COUNTS

About a decade ago, a group led by Peter Scardino, a respected expert on prostate cancer and former head of urology and surgery at Memorial Sloan-Kettering, and including Vickers, looked at how prostate cancer patients' outcomes correlated with the number of surgeries conducted by the doctors who treated them. Did the doctors' experience matter? They found that results of the surgery (as measured by cancer recurrence rates) improved substantially as the total number of prostatectomies performed by the patients' doctors increased, with this improvement eventually leveling off once the physicians hit around 250 career prostate surgeries.[13]

"We then thought, oh, well, how long does it take for the typical surgeon to get up that learning curve?" Vickers said. "So we did a study looking at what was the typical surgeon's volume in the U.S. per year."

The findings were not encouraging. The most common number of prostatectomies performed per year was one. The median number was three. Roughly 80 percent of physicians performing prostatectomies did fewer than 10 each year.[14] In other words, these surgeons did not have the extensive experience that, the researchers found, produced the best outcomes.

"These were general urologists," Vickers said. "So they would do their two radical prostatectomies per year and the rest of the time they would be doing kidney stones or bed wetting or erectile dysfunction. So we had evidence that your treatment strongly depended on whether you were getting surgery from an experienced surgeon. And huge numbers of patients were getting surgery from very inexperienced surgeons."

Doctors were using PSA testing indiscriminately; they were too quick to follow up the tests with biopsies; they were treating too many low-risk cancers with biopsies; and they were often inexperienced in conducting surgery or other treatments.

Vickers still believed, however, that there was a path forward. He analogized the state of PSA testing to that of car safety decades ago, when there were tens of thousands of fatalities from crashes every year. People didn't stop driving, though, Vickers noted. Instead, the government worked to make driving safer.

Scardino has developed recommendations on how to properly use the PSA test for cancer screening, showing just how many details are involved in doing it well.

As with any screening test, the first step is deciding who should be screened. According to Scardino, men should undergo their first PSA test sometime between ages 45 and 49. Assuming the test is normal (a score of less than 1 ng/ml at that age), the men should repeat testing every five years. If at age 60 they still have a score of less than 1 ng/ml, they can safely stop PSA screening.

"We're trying to increase screening in the younger population who has the most to benefit, and decrease it as a man gets older," Scardino said.

What, though, of men whose PSA tests come back higher than normal, indicating that they might have prostate cancer? He outlined a series of methodical steps.

Men with a PSA of between 1 and 3 should typically return every two years for testing, Scardino said. For individuals with a score between 3 and 10, additional analysis is needed to decide whether they should undergo a biopsy. The first thing Scardino recommends in the case of these patients is to wait and test again. In about 40 percent of such cases, a patient's high PSA score will drop back to normal levels on its own in around six to twelve weeks, he said.

If the second test confirms that the elevated PSA reading is real, Scardino said, he would then order additional blood- or urine-based testing, an MRI, or both, depending on how concerned he was based on indications from the PSA tests and digital rectal exams.

Such additional tests to further assess patients are known as reflex tests. Scardino and Vickers are codevelopers of a PSA reflex test called the 4Kscore, which measures the levels of four proteins, including PSA, to help determine whether a high test score truly indicates prostate cancer. Studies have found this reflex test could reduce unnecessary prostate biopsies by 30 percent to 58 percent.[15]

There are now several reflex tests available to evaluate high PSA scores and strike a better balance between overtreatment and under-treatment. Commonly used tests include the free-to-total PSA ratio, which measures two forms of PSA, and the Prostate Health Index, which measures three forms of the protein. In addition, many other PSA reflex tests are in various stages of development.

MRIs are another follow-up tool that can help doctors evaluate elevated PSA levels, though Scardino noted that false positive results are a challenge. Prostate MRI findings are reported using the Prostate Imaging Reporting & Data System (PI-RADS), which scores images on a scale of 1 to 5, where 1 indicates a very low chance that cancer is present and 5 indicates a very high chance that cancer is present. Patients with a PI-RADS score of 1 or 2 are generally not recommended for biopsy, while men with scores of 4 or 5 typically are. However, scores of 3 (which comprise 20 to 30 percent of prostate MRI results[16]) are more difficult to interpret, Scardino said, observing that only around 20 percent of these men will have clinically significant cancer (meaning a cancer requiring treatment).

One of the biggest shifts in prostate cancer care has been the increased reliance on active surveillance for managing tumors. Active surveillance refers to the practice of regularly monitoring men diagnosed with low to moderate risk prostate cancer instead of opting right away for surgery. This lets patients avoid the side effects of a prostatectomy while the doctors continue to measure PSA levels and monitor the growth rate of the tumors. Surgery or other interventions are considered if there are indications of rapid development of the cancer.

That approach has become an increasingly common strategy for dealing with prostate cancers, especially as concern has grown over the risk of overtreatment. While at one time just 5 percent to 10 percent of patients with low-risk cancers were managed with this type of careful monitoring, that figure has risen to about 50 percent today and it is above 90 percent at most of the leading medical centers, according to Vickers.

"Things are moving in the right direction," Vickers said. "The thing about PSA screening and the question of does 'it' work, or does 'it' do more good than harm, is that it's not an 'it,' it's not a single thing like 81 milligrams of aspirin. It's a whole package of things that have to be done together. Who do we screen? Who do we decide to biopsy? Who do we decide to treat? What treatment should they get? Who should be doing that treatment? If you do all that right, you have a very strong chance of doing a lot more good than harm."

THE MAMMOGRAM SCARE: POPULAR AND MISUSED FOR BREAST CANCER SCREENING

As PSA testing faced serious questions, another public controversy was developing around mammography, the popular early-detection tool for breast cancer in women. Aside from Pap smears, no other cancer screening tool is more consistently used by its target population than mammography, and probably none have achieved the same level of recognition and prominence. But concerns have been raised about the test's usefulness and accuracy due largely to false positives and questions about overdiagnosis and follow-up procedures.

Roughly one in eight women will develop breast cancer over their lifetime, making it the most common malignancy (aside from non-melanoma skin cancer) among women in the U.S. Over the last thirty years, breast cancer mortality rates have declined by more than 40 percent, with the uptake of screening mammography responsible for a substantial portion of that drop.[17] Mammography is far from a perfect tool, however.

To begin with, mammograms miss a fairly large portion of breast cancers—up to 25 percent—with many of those cancers being aggressive. Additionally, mammograms are less effective for the roughly 50 percent of women who have dense breast tissue—breasts with a high proportion of glandular and fibrous tissue that can mask the appearance of tumors. Further, many women are unaware of the test's flaws and downsides,[18] and thus face difficulty in understanding and responding to the results.

As with PSA, though, the answer isn't to stop screening. Clinical trials have consistently shown that mammography lowers breast cancer mortality to a significant degree. It is certainly a useful test. The question is if better follow-up procedures and new technologies can make it even more reliable.

The origins of screening mammography—a type of low-energy x-ray that can identify lumps and other abnormalities inside the tissue of breasts—go back to the 1950s when Jacob Gershon-Cohen, a radiologist at Philadelphia's Albert Einstein Medical Center, used the technique in a cohort of more than 1,000 healthy women, screening them regularly over five years. He identified twenty-three cancers, including six that couldn't be detected by a physical exam.[19]

The first large-scale RCT of screening mammography was launched in 1963, with 62,000 members of the Health Insurance Plan of Greater New York participating. The findings, released in 1971, showed that mammography was highly effective.[20] For women between 50 and 59, screening reduced breast cancer deaths by 40 percent. Since then, there have been nine additional RCTs studying mammography, all of which found a decrease in breast cancer mortality.

And yet, as we find in most cancer screening tests, the details on who should be tested, what to do about false positives, and how to provide testing equitably provide thorny complications. In the case of mammography, some are skeptical about the benefits—especially in younger women, and the 40–49 age cohort in particular. As Handel Reynolds, a radiologist, details in *The Big Squeeze*, his history of mammography, organizations including the NCI and the American Cancer Society have debated for decades whether women under 50 should undergo regular screening.[21]

In 2009, the U.S. Preventive Services Task Force sparked controversy when it declined to recommend regular mammograms for this population, reversing guidelines it had put in place in 2002. That same year, a commentary in *JAMA* (*The Journal of the American Medical Association*) by several high-profile physicians suggested that the medical community reevaluate its approach to breast cancer screening.[22]

At the heart of this skepticism was data showing that since the implementation of mammography programs, the number of cases of early-stage breast cancers had risen dramatically, but without an equivalent decline in the number of women with late-stage disease.[23] That has been interpreted to mean that many of the early-stage cancers that mammography is detecting might not have grown into late-stage tumors and would therefore never have threatened those women's lives. This was evidence of overdiagnosis, the skeptics argued.

Estimates of overdiagnosis vary widely, from as little as 1 percent of cases to more than 30 percent, but with many estimates falling in the 5 percent to 10 percent range.[24]

FALSE POSITIVES AND OVERTREATMENT

There is also a problem of mammography's high false positive rates. The false positive rate for an individual mammogram is about 10 percent, which is not generally regarded as an excessive figure by medical researchers. Women do not typically just stop with a single mammo-gram, however—they are screened annually or biennially for twenty years or more, and each screening presents an additional opportunity to receive a false positive result.

In the late 1990s, researchers calculated the chance that a woman undergoing regular mammograms would receive a false positive over a period of ten years. They arrived at a figure of 49 percent. Perhaps even more significantly, they projected that, after ten years of annual mammograms, 19 percent of women would undergo an unnecessary biopsy.

Those numbers came as a surprise even to some of the doctors leading the study. "I knew that it was going to be high, but even I was shocked that it was that high," said Joann Elmore, an internist at UCLA and first author on the *New England Journal of Medicine* paper that detailed the findings.[25]

While some level of false positives are regarded as inevitable, El-more suggested that the abbreviated nature of clinical trials—where individuals are typically screened only a handful of times—understat-ed the extent of the challenge. When women receive the test for many years, the potential for problems naturally grows.

"Most investigators in cancer screening don't think longitudinally like I do," she said. "People have data from randomized clinical trials where they may be screening people three times, five times. But can-cer screening is being recommended for three decades, and people need to realize that."

"I'm a primary care doctor. I take care of patients for decades," she added. "I see them coming back, and I see both the positives and neg-atives of cancer screening. So I've encouraged people to look at the cumulative outcome from screening."

In 2009, just under a decade after the *New England Journal of Medicine* paper was published, the U.S. Preventive Services Task Force, influenced by the work by Elmore and her colleagues, ruled not to recommend screening for women ages 40 to 49. It maintained that stance in a 2016 update of its guidelines.[26]

Studies have shown that starting mammography screening at age 40 slightly reduces breast cancer deaths compared to starting at age 50, but the lower incidence of breast cancer in women 40 to 49 and the higher incidence of false positives among this age group shifted the task force's thinking.

Recently the task force proposed returning to its pre-2009 recommendation that all women 40 years and older receive regular mammograms. In a draft guidance issued in May 2023, it said that "new and more inclusive science . . . now supports all women getting screened, every other year, starting at age 40."[27]

A major consideration driving the proposed recommendation is data indicating that starting screening at age 40 could be particularly beneficial for Black women, who, the Preventive Services Task Force draft report noted, have a "higher breast cancer mortality especially among younger" individuals.

The same tradeoff between breast cancers detected and false positives remains. The models cited in both the 2016 update and the 2023 draft guidelines show that starting screening at 40 versus 50 increases the number of breast cancer deaths prevented by roughly 1 per 1,000 women screened, while increasing the number of false positives by around 50 percent to 60 percent.

There's also a flipside to the false positive issue. Despite regular screening, some breast cancers still manage to avoid early detection. Roughly a quarter of breast cancers are what are known as interval cancers, meaning they develop and are diagnosed during the interval between a woman's mammograms. These cancers are also, on average, more aggressive than mammogram-detected tumors—and deadlier. In other words, the breast cancers that mammography is most likely to miss are, unfortunately, more threatening cancers.

"We're great at finding cancers that are slowly growing," said Victoria Seewaldt, an oncologist at City of Hope Comprehensive Cancer Center. "But we have a lot of aggressive cancers that we're not good at screening."

Part of the problem, Seewaldt said, is that mammography is not strong at detecting one of the deadliest classes of breast cancer, called triple-negative tumors. That means the tumor cells lack all three of the proteins—estrogen receptor, progesterone receptor, and human epidermal growth factor, or HER2—that are most vulnerable to and commonly targeted by breast cancer drugs. One of the main ways mammograms find tumors is by picking up calcifications, deposits of calcium in the breast that are sometimes associated with cancer. However, less than 15 percent of triple-negative cancers feature calcifications and so they can go undetected until later stages when they cause symptoms and can be more difficult to stop.

"I think mammography is a great tool," Seewaldt said. "If you're talking about some 40-year-olds and generally for 50 and above it works really, really well. But in young women who tend to get these rapidly growing, aggressive cancers that don't typically form calcifications, it's just the wrong tool for the job. And then we blame mammography when really the blame should go to the fact that we are not really using our heads."

There is also the issue of denser breast tissue. That tissue can hide tumors on a mammogram, decreasing the test's sensitivity. Studies have found that while mammograms detect between 86 percent and 89 percent of cancers in women with low breast density, that drops to between 62 percent and 68 percent in women with extremely dense breasts.[28]

While breast density typically decreases with age, roughly 50 percent of women have either dense or extremely dense breasts.[29] Growing awareness of this issue has led thirty-eight states and the District of Columbia to pass laws requiring healthcare providers to notify women about their breast density when reporting mammogram results. Eighteen states also require providers to inform women with dense breasts about supplemental screening methods, such as ultrasound, that may pick up tumors missed by mammography.

Additionally, the FDA is updating its mammography quality standards to include guidelines for reporting breast density information to patients so they can understand screening limitations. There are also efforts to require that insurers cover supplemental screening for women with dense breasts. In late 2022, Congress began considering a bill—the Find It Early Act—that would mandate such coverage.

It is uncertain, though, how much these moves will improve breast cancer outcomes. Breast density reporting laws appear to have produced an uptick in cancer detection, but only a modest one,[30] and this gain in sensitivity has been accompanied by an increase in false positives generated by the supplemental screening.[31] The ultimate costs and benefits of density-based breast cancer screening protocols thus remain unclear. The new U.S. Preventive Services Task Force draft guidelines do not recommend supplemental screening for women with dense breast tissue. According to the task force, "there is not yet enough evidence . . . to recommend for or against additional screening" for these women.

Further complicating the mammography issue is the growing detection of what is known as DCIS, or ductal carcinoma in situ. DCIS is a noninvasive form of breast cancer characterized by abnormal cells in a woman's milk duct. It is, fortunately, highly curable. But doctors have raised the question of when they really need to treat these cancers, and, if they do, what are the best treatments.

Like other carcinomas referred to as in situ, DCIS is sometimes labeled stage 0 cancer, which means that, though little developed, it may be a precursor to more invasive stages of the disease. A percentage of women with untreated DCIS will go on to develop invasive cancers, though the exact relationship between the original DCIS abnormality and the subsequent invasive tumor is not certain. Studies indicate that more than half of patients with untreated, high-grade DCIS will develop invasive breast cancer within five years. Somewhere between 35 percent and 50 percent of low-grade DCIS patients will ultimately develop an invasive breast cancer if left untreated, but over a period that can span decades.[32]

Additionally, research suggests that when low-grade DCIS does progress to invasive breast cancer, those cancers are commonly "lower-grade, slow-growing, and early-detectable" lesions "with excellent prognosis," according to a 2019 report in the *British Journal of Cancer*. [33]

"The presentation of DCIS is really different from invasive cancer," said Shelley Hwang, a surgical oncologist at the Duke Cancer Institute whose research focuses on these lesions. "DCIS rarely presents as a lump. It very rarely spreads to the lymph nodes. It almost seems like a completely different disease."

In theory, large percentages of DCIS patients could safely skip or postpone treatment for the condition—treatment that typically involves surgery. That could include a mastectomy for 20 percent to 30 percent of the patients, followed by radiation and hormone therapy.

Doctors currently have few tools to help them distinguish between the more threatening and less dangerous lesions. So the field has largely opted for an aggressive approach to treatment. That probably saves lives, but the problem is that while mammography is not very effective at detecting certain types of aggressive breast cancers, it is quite good at picking up cases of DCIS.

The result is what you would expect—there has been a sharp rise in cases as more women have undergone breast screening over the past several decades. Between 1983 and 2003, the number of detected DCIS cases increased by roughly 500 percent.[34] Today, between 20 percent and 25 percent of new breast cancer diagnoses are DCIS.

The situation, Hwang noted, is somewhat analogous to that faced in prostate cancer following the widespread adoption of PSA testing. Mammography identifies large numbers of low-risk lesions. The doctors send many women to treatment for cancers that might have never threatened their lives. With prostate cancer, there are many responses to positive tests short of major interventions. But that is less true for DCIS.

"I think in some ways it has been easier to move in prostate cancer because the downside of treatment is so significant," Hwang said. "It's harder for the medical community to deal with [the] psycho-social consequences" involved in treating DCIS. "But I think those are very real, and I'm sure I've done double mastectomies on patients with DCIS and really impacted their life and their quality of life forever."

With prostate cancer, RCTs have shown that low-risk cancers can be treated with surveillance without significantly increasing patient mortality.[35] But there have not been any similar trials for breast cancer to guide doctors and patients on alternative approaches. That should change. Several ongoing trials, including one led by Hwang, are assessing whether surveillance is a safe approach with low-risk DCIS. An answer is still years away, but such trials may help lift mammography's cost-benefit ratio in the right direction.

ONE FIX: STANDARDIZING PRACTICES FOR FOLLOW-UP PROCEDURES

There are hopeful indications that the false positive issue can be improved. One striking piece of information is that the false positive rates for mammography in the U.S. are significantly higher than in many other countries. When researchers with the Norwegian Breast Cancer Screening Program looked at the cumulative risk of receiving a false positive result over the course of 10 scans in that country, they arrived at 21 percent[36]—less than half the rate Elmore and her colleagues calculated for U.S. women. A similar study in Spain calculated a cumulative rate of 32 percent.[37] Those are indications that the U.S. can do better.

A key metric for tracking false positives is what is known as the recall rate—the percent of mammograms that are flagged for additional follow-up. The American College of Radiology recommends radiologists to maintain a mammography recall rate of between 5 percent and 12 percent. Rates below that 5 percent cutoff suggest that doctors may be missing cancers by not recalling enough borderline cases for further investigation. Recall rates of more than 12 percent, on the other hand, can be associated with unnecessarily high follow-up to false positives. A recent study of U.S. radiologists found that more than 40 percent had recall rates above the 12 percent threshold.[38]

Elizabeth Morris, a radiologist at the University of California, Davis, and an expert in breast imaging, suggested that the high rate of false positives in the U.S. reflects the lack of any centralized breast screening program or standardized guidelines.

"If you look at national screening programs like they have in Europe or throughout the rest of the world, they have expert screening readers, and they have benchmarks that you have to achieve in order to remain a reader in the program," she said.

That contrasts with the U.S., where many mammograms are interpreted by radiologists in private practice. Reading breast scans may be only a small part of their work. As with urologists and prostatectomies, radiologists get better the more mammograms they read. But while in other countries expert readers typically analyze several thousand mammograms per year, in the U.S. radiologists need to read only 480 mammograms annually to maintain accreditation.

"You don't build up a lot of experience reading that few mammograms," Morris said. "I think it's horrendous [the minimum standard] is that low."

She suggested that, in an ideal world, screening mammograms would be read by groups of expert readers, much as they are in other countries with standardized screening practices. She noted that the rise of telehealth radiology technologies, which allow for easier sharing of imaging, should make the prospect of developing teams of expert readers with greater levels of experience feasible.

Morris said that she and others who share her views have lobbied to increase the requirements for readers but had found little appetite for such initiatives at professional organizations like the American College of Radiology.

"They don't want to do that because most of their constituents are private practitioners, and it would be really hard [if annual reading requirements were increased] for private practitioners to qualify their people to be mammography readers."

New mammography technologies might help alleviate the problems. These include digital breast tomosynthesis, known as DBT, which produces a sort of 3D mammogram. Introduced roughly a decade ago, DBT computers combine multiple breast x-rays to create a three-dimensional model of a patient's breasts. DBT is widely available, making up around 30 percent of mammography instruments in the U.S., and are in operation at roughly 80 percent of the country's mammography facilities.[39] Around half of the mammograms performed in the U.S. are now done using DBT.

This is likely to prove a favorable development. A number of studies have found that, compared to the previous generation of 2D mammograms, DBT improves detection of cancers while also lowering both false positives and recall rates.[40] The NCI is currently supporting a 165,000-women RCT comparing the two approaches. The study is scheduled to finish in 2030. But given the rapid pace of adoption even without evidence from a large trial, it seems likely that DBT will become the de facto standard of care before the study is concluded and the findings reported.

MRIs can also help detect breast cancers missed by mammography, though they are primarily used to supplement conventional mammographic screening in women with family histories or genetic mutations that put them at high risk for the disease. While MRIs can pick up small tumors undetectable by mammograms, they are less effective at detecting the microcalcifications that are common signs of breast cancer. Additionally, breast MRIs produce significantly more false positive findings than mammography, with some studies indicating a nearly sixfold higher false positive rate for MRIs[41].

Morris of UC Davis is a proponent of another advanced technology—contrast enhanced digital mammography, or CEDM—that has also been shown to reduce false positives while enhancing tumor detection. CEDM uses a contrast dye, which highlights various features inside the breast tissue, making it easier for the radiologist to identify and evaluate suspicious abnormalities.

CEDM has largely been tested as a tool for screening high-risk women. That is a category that consists primarily of women known or suspected of carrying certain genetic characteristics that increase their vulnerability to malignancies. But Morris believes that CEDM could be useful to a broader set of women, including average-risk women and women with denser breast tissue, with improved results.

One potential challenge to expanding use of CEDM is that the iodine-based contrast agents used by the technique can have side effects in some patients. These effects range from mild allergic reactions to conditions like contrast-induced nephropathy that can be life threatening. They are rare, but even low prevalence side-effects can be cause for concern when extrapolated over a population-scale screening cohort. This is also an issue for the gadolinium dye commonly used in breast MRIs, which, according to some experts, could have long-term impacts on brain health.

Cancer screening will always require compromises. Sensitivity, specificity, and side effects will exist in tension with each other. The goal, of course, is to refine screening protocols so that patients receive the maximum benefits with the minimum downside risk and to remain focused on the overall benefits, the lives saved by early detection.

ENDING THE ONE-SIZE-FITS-ALL APPROACH TO BREAST CANCER SCREENING

A study led by researchers at the University of California, San Francisco, is exploring the issue of how doctors can balance those many factors.

It is called the WISDOM study, for Women Informed to Screen Depending On Measures of risk, and it aims to recruit about 70,000 women to participate. They will be divided into two groups—a control arm in which all women will receive annual mammograms and an experimental arm in which participants will be screened according to individual risk assessments that will include medical and family histories as well as genetic testing for mutations and variants linked to breast cancer. Women in the experimental arm determined to be at low risk will be screened according to current U.S. Preventive Services Task Force guidelines. Those found to be at higher risk will receive more intensive screening, including and up to alternating mammograms and MRIs every six months.

The project grew out of work by the ATHENA Breast Care Network, an organization comprising five University of California medical centers that is following roughly 150,000 women over several decades. It is collecting personal and medical information that can be used to inform the development of better targeted prevention, screening, and treatment for breast cancer.

"The goal of the network is to bring together experts across the University of California system . . . to see how we can better evaluate every woman coming through the door and getting a mammogram to try to understand who is at risk, and for those who are at higher risk how we can intervene and offer them additional services," said Allison Fiscalini, director of the ATHENA Network and the WISDOM study.

Given the heterogeneity of the many types of breast cancer and the differences in risk profiles among women, "we think that a one-size-fits-all, aged-based screening recommendation is likely not the best recommendation for how to screen women," she commented. "That said, in order to actually test that and prove that, we had to and are doing a big screening trial to be able to provide prospective and randomized data to help answer this question."

The most immediate goal, Fiscalini said, is to make sure women with elevated breast cancer risk are provided with more intensive screening and, if appropriate, risk-reducing treatments like endocrine therapy or prophylactic mastectomies. A secondary aim would be to determine whether screening guidelines can be safely reduced for low-risk women.

Disseminating the benefits of the study's findings—assuming its risk-based approach does show an improvement over current breast cancer prevention, detection and mortality levels—will also be a challenge.

"There's a baseline-level knowledge that most providers have, but many of them are not trained to do a more in-depth risk assessment that fills in the nuances of the knowledge that we have around breast cancer risk assessment," Fiscalini said.

In fact, many providers aren't even putting that baseline-level knowledge to use. Nearly half of women do not currently discuss their known breast cancer risk factors with their doctors when contemplating or planning screening.[41] A program would need to be developed to ensure some level of dissemination of the findings of the WISDOM study and any recommendations. If necessary, there should be training for physicians and technicians so they can implement newly developed best practices.

The first step, though, is showing that it can work—demonstrating that things like better management of false positives and follow-up treatment, more thorough and widespread use of risk assessment, and more nuanced approaches to ductal carcinoma in situ, the noninvasive form of breast cancer, can inform mammography standards where the pros clearly outweigh the cons, particularly for younger women at lower risk. As Memorial Sloan-Kettering's Vickers puts it, the point of screening isn't "just to say, 'Well, it's got harms, it's got benefits, the benefits don't much outweigh the harms, and there you go.' No. Let's reduce the harms, and then the tradeoff is much easier."

CHAPTER 5
FROM SCREENING TO TREATMENT:

GETTING THE EARLY-DETECTION MESSAGE TO AT-RISK POPULATIONS

IT WAS LATE 2019 AND TIME TO TRY SOMETHING NEW.

Lung cancer has for years been our country's worst cancer killer, taking more than 130,000 lives every year. But the real news is that, though we know how to detect and, in many cases, stop this terrible disease by diagnosing it in its earliest stages with a simple test, shockingly few of those at risk take advantage of this technology. It's a story repeated throughout our battles with cancer, but it is particularly upsetting to consider how this affects lung cancer mortality rates, with too many early deaths.

The National Lung Screening Trial a decade ago demonstrated the effectiveness of the test, low-dose computed tomography, or LDCT, for detecting even very small tumors in the lungs, yet only about 4.5 percent of the at-risk population—smokers and former smokers—is getting the test. As a result of that poor uptake, only 3 percent of lung cancers are detected through screening, as opposed to through the emergence of symptoms, according to a study by NORC at the University of Chicago, a large independent data research institute.

By the time symptoms surface, lung cancer is often advanced, difficult to treat, and far more lethal. That is true of cancers generally. According to the study by NORC, a paltry 14.1 percent of Americans diagnosed with cancer learned that they had the disease through recommended early-detection screening tests.[1]

At the end of 2019, we planned and started our "something new": an experimental pilot program to try to turn the poor lung screening record around. The Michael D. Ratner Center for Early Detection of Cancer, a nonprofit founded by Bruce in memory of his late brother, partnered with physicians at New York's Weill Cornell Medicine on the pioneering project. The plan was to create a mobile lung screening unit with an LDCT device and have it offer tests in a medically under-served New York City neighborhood. If at-risk residents of the community were not going to medical centers for the screening perhaps, the thinking went, they might be willing to take the test, for free, right in their neighborhood.

A mobile unit was prepared and taken to the MetroTech Center, a large office complex in Brooklyn, chosen for its proximity to public transportation and a sizable population of medically underserved residents. The project targeted the at-risk individuals we wanted to reach through messages on social media and local radio and TV advertising, providing information and urging them to take advantage of this free service. And then we waited for the results.

The pilot's performance delivered a double-edged lesson, partly disappointing but ultimately providing hints of the successful path policymakers should pursue. In a little under a month, the partnership with Weill Cornell Medicine screened 216 people and identified 25 with possible cancer indications. After further testing and analysis, 2 of those 25 individuals were diagnosed with lung cancer, both stage IIB, and both patients underwent surgery to remove the tumors. Those are exactly the kinds of cancer patients healthcare providers want to identify at such an early stage.

But as we studied the results of our pilot, we discovered something unexpected. Of the forty-three patients who provided zip codes when surveyed, no one listed the zip code where the mobile van was parked. The closest were three people who came from adjacent zip codes. The whole strategy behind the pilot was to bring the screening equipment to people who needed it in an underserved neighborhood, but it did not appear that many of those in the imme-diate vicinity responded.

But we analyzed the data further and discerned another positive outcome from our experiment: it proved the value of mass media in reaching targeted audiences and conveying persuasive information about the need for and benefits of screening. Marketing today is, of course, a highly technical science, and we know that science works for all kinds of consumer products, from household cleaning supplies to soda, beer, and automobiles. The people who were willing to travel some way for the lung cancer screening were demonstrating the effectiveness of those marketing techniques for our pilot.

That was a useful lesson. Among the impediments to improving performance in the overall early-detection effort are a lack of research funding, the costs, patient indifference and fears, and a lack of public information reaching the people who need it most. It is increasingly clear that a critical missing ingredient is the application of sophisticated, comprehensive marketing and media campaigns. This concept has been proven in the healthcare field but its application is too rare. Perhaps the best examples of how this can work in practice are the CDC's Screen for Life campaign to increase colorectal screening and its "Tips" anti-smoking campaign.

The Tips campaign, formally called "Tips from Former Smokers," was started in 2012 and used very graphic, sobering, and sad testimonials from former smokers who had suffered terrible damage to their health from cigarettes. As in any commercial marketing campaign, there was a significant degree of audience testing and focus groups to shape the messages and measure results. The program's designers learned that most people were familiar with the lethal dangers of cigarettes as well as secondhand smoke but that was generally not enough to influence them to quit or avoid getting addicted in the first place. But seeing in the TV ads people disfigured by surgery to remove tumors or struggling to breathe and survive the disease's chronic, long-term impact, particularly how that affected their families, began to motivate smokers to take action.

Those emotional advertisements included information on how smokers could quit, directed them to smoking cessation programs and focused partly on ensuring that these messages reached underserved and low-income communities. In that way, the program contributed to addressing the disparities in smoking and lung cancer rates between those groups. The CDC estimates that, between 2012 and 2018, more than 16.4 million smokers who saw these ads tried to break their addictions to cigarettes, with about one million succeeding.

Those public service ads are not alone in proving the power of mass media, and television especially, to spread positive messages and influence behavior. Think about iconic slogans such as "Friends Don't Let Friends Drive Drunk" (anti-drunk driving), "You Can Learn a Lot from a Dummy" (encouraging drivers to wear seatbelts), and "Keep America Beautiful" (anti-littering and community improvement) from previous public service campaigns. We should be adding lung cancer screening to that list of successes. Such campaigns could transform screening participation.

Reaching medically underserved populations with cancer screening is a persistent challenge. Large gaps exist in screening and treatment rates between white and nonwhite populations, upper-income and lower-income populations, and urban and rural populations. Each disparity requires a significant, thoughtful effort to correct, but each successful step would translate into many thousands of lives saved every year from needless early deaths.

For instance, overall rates of colorectal and breast cancer screening are considerably higher than for lung cancer, but there are yawning disparities between different groups. In some parts of the country, compliance rates for breast and colorectal screening reach into the 90 percent range, while in others they remain as low as 30 percent.

One particularly illustrative example of the problem: researchers from the American Cancer Society found that before the introduction of widespread colorectal cancer screening, Black Americans had a lower colorectal cancer death rate than white Americans. After colorectal screening became more commonplace, those figures flipped, with Black Americans suffering higher death rates from the disease.[2]

Why? Screening led to more early detection of the disease, when it is curable, and white Americans generally received more screening, more treatment, and higher quality treatment than Black patients.

OVERCOMING THE CHALLENGE OF SCREENING EQUITY

Even though we know that targeted use of mass media campaigns could make significant contributions to solving this problem, the question of why some resist getting screened is complex and, often, there are no certain answers, just challenging experiences and anecdotes that hint at the underlying issues.

Maria Fernandez, director of the Center for Health Promotion and Prevention Research at the University of Texas Health Science Center, has been working for decades to boost cancer screening in Latino communities along the Texas-Mexico border, where screening rates are among the lowest in the United States. In her work on colorectal cancer, Fernandez has found that only about a quarter of this population is up to date on screening for the disease. Forty percent of the people in those communities aren't even aware that screening tests for colorectal cancer exist.[3]

Fernandez first became interested in cancer screening while a doctoral student at the University of Maryland in the 1990s. "I was working with a nonprofit that did education and provided services to immigrant populations, which in that area at that time was primarily Salvadoran," she recalled. She was interested in chronic disease prevention and particularly screening, "so I started working with that population, and for my doctoral dissertation developed an intervention to increase breast and cervical cancer screening."

For the past decade, Fernandez has been working in and around El Paso to improve access to screening for these two cancers among medically underserved women. Over that time, she and her team managed to get about half of those who went untested into screening.

"We've done a good job, right?" she said. "But as good as that is, it still leaves 50 percent consistently unscreened."

In part, this is a straightforward matter of resources. Access to healthcare is a constant problem in sparsely populated areas like the Texas border region. In fact, while racial and economic outcome disparities have been narrowing, the gap between people living in rural versus urban or suburban areas has been widening.

"Our [rural] counties are just emptying out and hospitals are going under," said Victoria Seewaldt of the City of Hope. "Say you have a breast mass, what are you going to do? You've got to travel 200 miles to maybe a nurse practitioner where you don't have an imaging center, you don't have high-quality imaging. And so you're just going to stay home."

To address the issue, Fernandez is involved in a project targeting rural residents for better screening access. She and her colleagues plan to provide self-sampling mail-in kits for cervical and colorectal cancer testing as well as for hepatitis, a major cause of liver cancer.

"It's an attempt to get those people who would otherwise not go to the clinic," she said, noting that while patients with positive findings would need to go to a clinic for follow-up testing, this would be a much smaller number. "So you could use more intensive resources to get those people" to a facility, "rather than use all of your resources to get the general population [to a clinic] when the majority of them would not be in need."

Fernandez said that the self-sampling campaign has received an enthusiastic response thus far. "The women just loved the idea," she said. "They thought, 'This is fantastic. I don't have to take off work. I can do it myself and mail it in. This is great.' They immediately saw it as a fantastic benefit."

Yet while access and resources are important, they are only part of the problem. There is fear, distrust, and other personal constraints.

"There is this belief that if you build it, they will come," Fernandez said. "And we know that that isn't true. Knowledge [alone] doesn't change behavior. Access is a necessary but not sufficient factor that influences screening."

Even her self-sampling project must battle subtle social constraints, she said. In previous work with Latino communities along the Texas-Mexico border, Fernandez and her colleagues found that men, in particular, associated cervical cancer with promiscuity, a linkage that they suggested could lead their female partners and relatives to avoid the screening.

Lung cancer screening runs into those often-silent complexities and barriers. For starters, researchers working to drive the adoption of LDCT will often say that one major barrier is the societal stigma surrounding cigarette smoking, the primary cause of lung cancer. People frequently feel shame about being or having been addicted to cigarettes, and that can make them less likely to seek out lung screening, which means confronting that shame.

Jamie Studts, a professor at the University of Colorado who has studied the factors people weigh when considering lung cancer screening, is working with the Bristol Myers Squibb Foundation and the LUNGevity Foundation, a nonprofit that seeks improved lung cancer treatments, to find better ways to engage people who are eligible for and should be getting the tests. Like Fernandez, he noted that the challenge goes beyond simply arming those people with the facts.

"There are a lot of times where we just sort of check the box for information delivery," he said. What's really needed are ways to "reach people, decrease the stigma barrier, and really engage them so that they start to have a positive feeling about the screening program."

There's no one silver bullet to removing the psychological barriers to screening, Studts said. But some common elements to approaches have demonstrated success.

One is peer pressure. In studying cervical cancer screening in Latina women, Fernandez found that one of the most significant factors in whether women get a Pap smear is if they believe their friends and family think they should.[4]

Connection, then—both to family and the larger community—seems to be at least one positive factor in persuading people to actively seek healthy practices and get the information they need.

THE PERSISTENCE NEEDED TO DRIVE HOME THE EARLY-DETECTION MESSAGE

One organization that has grappled with the early-detection challenge is the Susan G. Komen Foundation, a prominent breast cancer nonprofit. One of its objectives is persuading women to get recommended mammograms, even if those tests are acknowledged to have some flaws. About a decade ago during a Congressional hearing on cancer screening, Shelley Fuld Nasso, the organization's director of public policy, related the experience of a Komen-funded outreach worker in Mississippi that illustrated how difficult this can be.

The worker, Dorothy Julius, was trying to get a member of her church to schedule a mammogram. The woman, who was 46, was in a high-risk category; her mother and three of her sisters had died of breast cancer. But she told Julius that even if she did have breast cancer, she would rather not know. Over six months, Julius slowly worked to convince her, primarily through contacts at their church, to see a doctor for a screening. She finally did and, happily, received a normal test result.[5]

As Fernandez of the University of Texas said, successful cancer screening is far more complicated than "build it, and they will come."

THE SCIENCE OF GETTING SCREENING RIGHT

Implementation science is a dedicated field of study that attempts to find ways the medical community can address these barriers. The NCI began funding research into the field in 2000. David Chambers, the institute's deputy director for implementation science, said the effort was a product of policymakers' finally facing the harsh reality that they were faltering in delivering the promise of early-detection screening.

"If we don't translate all of the understanding we've amassed in terms of trying to get population level screening and prevention and health promotion, we aren't going to do much of a job of reducing the overall burden of cancer," he said.

The issue is translation—translating good science and effective tests into lower mortality rates.

"There was a lot of concern that we had spent all this money on cancer, and what did we have to show for it?" said Karen Emmons of Harvard's T.H. Chan School of Public Health. "And a lot of that is around the failure to move things into practice and translation. We built these things, but nobody is using them. Why is that? It's because we haven't thought about the patient space, and we developed these interventions that were kind of impractical. So, how do you start to develop them in different ways?"

Even though uptake is recognized as a critical issue, the NCI still provides only modest funding for implementation research. In 2015, researchers, including Chambers, tallied up the grant money NCI had provided for implementation science research projects between 2000 and 2012. They found that it had funded sixty-seven grants totaling about $93 million during that time, or slightly less than $8 million per year.[6] But the NCI's total annual research budget averaged between $4.5 billion and $5 billion during this period, dwarfing the funds for implementation and raising questions about how serious it is about breaking the logjam of disappointing early-detection use.

In 2019, the NCI launched its Implementation Science Centers in Cancer Control, or ISC3, initiative, a five-year program that provides funding to eight research centers around the country for cancer implementation studies. Again, though, the funding for the potentially significant program is relatively modest—about $8 million per year.[7] And that is still not money being invested in thoughtful TV and other proven targeted media programs.

A tricky aspect of these efforts is confronting the emotions and fears people have about cancer and screening, or using those emotions to enhance uptake, like the successful Tips anti-smoking program.

Some of these studies utilize a longstanding theory of patient behavior called the Health Belief Model. It was developed in the 1950s by Godfrey Hochbaum, a social psychologist working for the U.S. Public Health Services who was trying to understand why more people weren't taking advantage of free tuberculosis screenings, which were being offered across the country through mobile x-ray units. In studying attitudes, Hochbaum found that people's use of health interventions was determined, first, by their perceptions of the seriousness of the disease and, second, by how effective they believed the intervention would be at reducing the risk.

Hochbaum published a paper in 1956 laying out the conceptual framework behind the belief model, which he and others would continue to refine in the following years. Today, it remains one of the most commonly used tools for studying and planning healthcare interventions. And our understanding has improved with new approaches. The Theory of Planned Behavior, for instance, developed by Icek Ajzen, a psychologist at the University of Massachusetts, looks at the role of personal relationships and social norms in driving behavior toward medical screening.

The insights in these models have been deployed to varying degrees in efforts to increase adoption of early-detection screening. But their utility depends on factors such as how the insights inform the communications to those who need this information, how the message is tailored to different groups of people, and the means used to deliver the information to ensure that it reaches those who need it most.

"So much of what happens in practice and what happens in the community is influenced by how information is shared, how it's received, how it is sought, the different media channels through which people are in some cases learning about the best possible practice, and in other cases about things that might actually not be all that helpful," said Chambers.

The basic notion underpinning implementation is that there must be convincing, easily understandable data, as well as an emotional dimension, to demonstrate the effectiveness of the screening tests. It is also important to have the supportive approval of a responsible government body to provide a sense of authoritative affirmation and credibility that the public can understand. Just as there is a government body that determines what cancer screenings and other preventive treatments to recommend—the U.S. Preventive Services Task Force—there is an organization that evaluates, approves, and promotes the most effective evidence-based implementation interventions: The Guide to Community Preventive Services.

THE COMMUNITY GUIDE: AN IMPLEMENTATION TOOL HIDING IN PLAIN SIGHT

The Community Guide, as it is known, was established in 1996 by the U.S. Department of Health and Human Services, and the group that produces it is housed within the CDC. Since its launch, it has produced about 250 recommendations, including many for cancer screenings. In 2019, for instance, it recommended the use of community health workers to directly encourage greater adoption of breast, cervical, and colorectal cancer screenings.

The guide has recommended approaches like one-on-one patient education, automated patient reminders, and reducing out-of-pocket costs. The implementation guide is regarded as the most comprehensive and well-researched assessment of what works best in getting people to embrace medical interventions, including cancer screening.

Putting that knowledge to work is easier said than done. Medical professionals must strike an appropriate balance between fidelity to evidence-based implementation models that have been analyzed and tested, and flexibility so that the models can be adapted to different communities or groups.

Those are challenging issues for the experts to work with. But the sad reality is that even the best-designed implementation strategies often sit on a shelf or face endless trials and are not put into practice in the real world. They are nothing more than academic research subjects, unfortunate symbols of the lack of attention paid to policies that make sure targeted population groups enjoy the potentially lifesaving benefits of early-detection technologies and follow-up treatment. They are also a testament to the unfortunate lack of well-crafted mass media campaigns to ensure that at-risk populations receive needed screening information in hard-hitting and persuasive ways, perhaps every time they switch on their TVs.

Even in cases where evidence-based models are used, there is often insufficient follow-up to maintain the programs with consistent energy. In 2012, the CDC began encouraging the sites it funded to use combinations of five intervention models aimed at boosting levels of breast and cervical cancer screening. Three of the models targeted patients and two targeted healthcare providers to improve their implementation practices. A few years later, researchers from the agency assessed usage. They measured uptake among the sixty-seven grantees (comprising fifty states, the District of Columbia, five U.S. territories, and eleven tribes or tribal organizations) from July 2012 to June 2013 and then between July 2014 and June 2015.

At baseline, all sixty-seven grantees reported use of at least three of the five interventions. Thirty reported using all five for an overall average of 4.1 intervention models.[8] But two years later, those figures had fallen to twenty-three grantees using all five intervention models and an overall average for use of 3.8.[9]

THE FUNDING BARRIER

The CDC researchers did not explore why usage rates for the screening programs had dropped among the grantees, but work by Ross Brownson, a professor of public health at Washington University in St. Louis, suggests that, in many cases, public health interventions are discontinued for reasons having nothing to do with their effectiveness. It is often money.

Brownson has focused some of his research on what is known as misimplementation, a phenomenon in public health where either effective interventions that should continue are ended, or ineffective interventions that should be ended continue. In 2015, Brownson and some colleagues published a study in the American Journal of Preventive Medicine surveying public health professionals around the country about how frequently they observed program misimplementation.[10]

Of the 944 public health workers interviewed, 39 percent said their department or agency had ended interventions that, judged by their effectiveness, should have been continued. Cancer programs were less likely to be halted inappropriately than other kinds of interventions, but 28 percent of respondents said that their organizations had ended beneficial cancer interventions.

Funding was often the deciding factor. More than 80 percent of respondents said the end of grant funding was one of the most common reasons for shutting down a successful program; more than 60 percent said funding had been shifted to a different intervention. These kinds of funding challenges, Brownson said, are simply a fact of life, especially for smaller local health initiatives.

"State health departments tend to have more steady streams of funding," he said. "Local health departments might have some local revenue, but they are often dependent on writing grants to various agencies, often the state health department."

Brownson is working under a five-year grant from NIH to develop a deeper understanding of the misimplementation issues. He and his colleagues are looking at the factors involved in launching and sustaining public health interventions to identify the critical pivot points that determine whether a program is successful and will be maintained.

"By modeling this, what we hope to have is sort of a cookbook for public health leaders to say, if you want to do something about this, here are what look like two or three of the key leverage points where you can really make a difference and make better use of the public health resources you are trying to put towards this problem in cancer or other areas," he said.

THE SCREEN FOR LIFE MODEL

A good example of what has worked well is the CDC's Screen for Life initiative, one of the most successful cancer screening programs and a model that should be emulated with other types of cancer screening—particularly its use of effective advertising and marketing. The program was launched in 1999 to increase colorectal cancer testing, usually through colonoscopies. Between 2000 and 2019, the percentage of U.S. residents up to date with recommended colorectal cancer screenings nearly doubled, to more than two-thirds of the population, from about one-third.[11] What was the result? The colorectal cancer death rate almost halved during that time, falling to 12.8 per 100,000 population from 20.7 per 100,000 people,[12] indicating that more than 100,000 deaths from this disease may have been prevented.

When you look at how Screen for Life has been conducted, three things distinguish it—mass media, money, and time. Since it started two decades ago, the program has run more than $300 million worth of TV, radio, and print ads (most of that donated as public service announcements) across 3,500 outlets, generating more than 20 billion impressions from the audiences. It has generated approximately 360 million online ad impressions and used more than 225 focus groups in dozens of cities around the country to test and refine its messaging. That is exactly the kind of media market saturation that is essential for success.

The program's messaging is concerted and extensive. Its television spots run on more than 1,000 networks nationwide, while its radio ads run on some 1,200 stations, and its print advertisements run in 2,000 magazines and 6,000 newspapers. It produces posters, videos, and other displays for out-of-home advertising in places like airports, shopping centers, public transit hubs, and even building elevators. It delivers educational and promotional materials to local partners around the country customized for their specific markets and populations.

By the standards of cancer screening outreach, Screen for Life has been a colossal effort and, as a result, exceptionally effective.[13] It has also been an enduring one. The program, which has enjoyed steady funding, has been able to move carefully and deliberately, allowing major returns on the resources deployed.

For instance, before the initiative was even formally launched, CDC scientists conducted fourteen focus groups at sites in Atlanta, Philadelphia, and Overland Park, Kansas, to learn what people knew and how they felt about colorectal cancer and colorectal cancer screening.[14] The scientists found a broad lack of awareness around the disease and screening and especially around the idea that screening could actually help doctors prevent colorectal cancer.

That finding suggested that an initial goal of programs should be to inform the public about the disease and the availability of screening, an effort to make that understanding commonplace. Communicating basic facts about colorectal cancer would also, it was hoped, make people more comfortable discussing it with peers, family members, and their doctors, and make them seek out and be comfortable with screening recommendations.

Once launched, the CDC researchers continued to run focus groups, enabling them to adjust the approach as public awareness deepened. During the first four years of the project, they conducted more than seventy focus groups in thirty cities around the U.S.[15] Over time, they realized, they were achieving the first goal of basic awareness and so prepared for the next phase of the campaign, providing more detailed information about the different colorectal cancer screening tests and how they work. The publicity materials were regularly updated to reflect the new messaging.

The program has continued this step-by-step approach for two decades, periodically evaluating its messaging and revising it in response to the targeted population's growing understanding.

Getting the messages to the right audiences and persuading them to listen has meant leaving the world of public health and diving into the advertising business. What factors, for instance, determine whether a broadcaster is likely to choose your public service announcement for free airtime? How do you contact and enlist celebrity spokespeople to spread your message—a tactic on which Screen for Life has relied heavily—and which figures are most likely to resonate with your audience? CDC staff collect such data from across all the country's 210 TV markets.[16]

Screen for Life is a positive story of the medical community's embracing modern marketing strategies to improve adoption of early-detection testing. But there is, unfortunately, another less salutary lesson—that the funding made available for cancer screening campaigns is, in truth, paltry. Screen for Life gets a particularly big bang for its advertising bucks because of the donated time it receives in the form of public service announcements. Its actual government advertising budget is only about $1 million a year. By contrast, the Big Pharma companies—who are competing with the government for the attention of consumers—spend sizable multiples of that modest sum on their drugs.

How much more? In 2020, for example, Bristol Myers Squibb spent $164.8 million on TV spots for a single cancer therapy, its Opdivo (+ Yervoy) immunotherapy regimen.[17] Even comparing that against Screen for Life's donated advertising, Bristol Myers Squibb still spent in a single year more than half the overall value of the CDC campaign in more than two decades. And that's just for Bristol Myers Squibb's television advertising, which, for the pharma industry in general, has made up around three-quarters of its marketing budget.[18]

Of course, the dollars spent were related to the dollars earned. Bristol Myers Squibb sold $8.7 billion worth of Opdivo and Yervoy in 2020.[19] With that kind of revenue, it's reasonable that the company would spend more than $150 million on TV spots. Colonoscopies, on the other hand, generate well over $1 billion a year in billings, but this money doesn't go to a single private entity. It is dispersed throughout the thousands of hospitals, clinics, technicians, and gastroenterologists involved in performing the procedures.

In the case of Opdivo (+ Yervoy), the advertising supports sales of a treatment that, while helpful for some patients, does vastly less to reduce cancer death rates than colorectal cancer screening.

The response of some experts is that pharma companies, motivated by profit potential, have far more reason to throw such huge sums into advertising compared with early-detection screening, which produces far less revenue. Meanwhile, many public health departments battle for grants to keep their modest early-detection outreach efforts alive. As we discuss in a later chapter, some promising new blood-based cancer screening tests that could be transformative are being developed for the market by private companies, including Exact and GRAIL, and those commercial prospects may well produce strong funding streams for marketing.

Only policymakers willing to invest in and eager to correct the medical system's early-detection shortcomings can rethink the spending priorities and start to generate improvements in the disappointing efforts to reduce cancer deaths.

CHAPTER 6

PATIENT NAVIGATORS TRANSFORM CANCER CARE

IN THE EARLY 1970S, HAROLD P. FREEMAN, A YOUNG AFRICAN American surgeon at New York's Harlem Hospital assigned to the breast clinic, noticed an unwelcome trend—a large percentage of his patients were being diagnosed with very advanced cancers, the hardest to treat, and thus were experiencing high mortality rates. Troubled by the development, Freeman set out to learn why so many women were coming to him only once it was too late to stop the malignancies.

In a sense, it was just the kind of opportunity to make a real difference that Freeman had been waiting for. He was raised in the Columbia Heights neighborhood of Washington, D.C., attended Catholic University, and then studied medicine at the Howard University Medical School. At Howard he came under the tutelage of Jack White and LaSalle Leffall, pioneering cancer surgeons, both of whom had trained at Memorial Sloan-Kettering Cancer Center in New York. (White was the first African American doctor to train in surgical oncology at Sloan-Kettering.)

The pair encouraged Freeman to do a year of his general surgical residency at Memorial Sloan-Kettering. He followed that with three more years as a senior resident there studying surgical oncology. Freeman finished his residency in 1967, finding himself, as he described it, "at the top of my field in [terms of] training," and trying to decide what to do next. Returning to Howard was an obvious option, but with White and Leffall already on staff there, he felt his expertise would be redundant. He went to work in Harlem instead.

Freeman grew up in a family of professionals—his father was a lawyer and his grandfather was a doctor who had also studied at the Howard Medical School half a century before him. But his father had died young, of testicular cancer, when Freeman was just 13, leaving his mother, a schoolteacher, with the challenge of raising him and his two brothers.

"We had connections to people who were educated, but my family didn't have money," he said.

Additionally, Washington, D.C., was a highly segregated city. And while Freeman thought little about it at the time, this upbringing laid the foundation for what would become an enduring interest in what he termed the social justice aspects of medicine, an interest that led him to stay in New York and to focus on more equitable healthcare for lower-income communities.

"I wanted to work in a poor Black community," he said. "I could have gone back to Washington, but I decided that I wanted to go to Harlem because I thought I would have an opportunity to do things that hadn't been done at Harlem Hospital."

It was there, as a young attending physician, that Freeman realized that by the time many of his patients saw him, their cancers were so advanced that there was little he could do.

The patients didn't have small tumors that had simply gone unnoticed. In some women, their cancers had progressed so far as to become ulcerated, causing open wounds. These were precisely the kinds of people Freeman was inspired to help, but he had to try to learn why they were delaying treatment so long in the effort to remedy the situation. As a first step, he interviewed them.

"I called a number of them in to talk to them while they were still alive, to ask them, 'Why did you come in so late?'" he said. "And they told me the story of what had actually led to it."

Many of them were single women with children and said they had actually come to the hospital emergency room years earlier after finding worrisome lumps in their breasts. That, it turned out, just led to a gauntlet of challenges in trying to obtain diagnoses and appropriate treatment, beginning with usually being told, after waiting hours to see a doctor, that they had come to the wrong place.

"You're in the emergency room," the women were told, as Freeman related the experiences. "And, you know, you have a lump in your breast, and that's not an emergency."

But before they could see a specialist for their care, they needed health insurance, which few had. So they were told to go to the Medicaid office, apply for and get an insurance card, then return to the hospital and make an appointment—not at the emergency room, but at the breast clinic.

Making this process even more onerous, the Medicaid office was some hundred blocks, about five miles, south of Harlem Hospital, a potentially time-consuming trip on public transportation.

"So you're asking a woman to go downtown, get an insurance card, come back, make a new appointment," Freeman said. "And these women, they were in tough circumstances. They were worried about food, shelter, avoiding crime, they had a lump in their breast. . . . Now they wait five hours to see a doctor, and he tells them to go downtown and come back with a card. What was being recommended to those women was more painful than what they thought they had."

A FREE CLINIC
SAVING LIVES

Freeman continued his interviews with the women over several years in the mid-1970s. When, toward the end of the decade, he was promoted to director of surgery at Harlem Hospital, he decided to use his new authority to develop strategies for tackling the problem. To start, he won a $25,000 grant from the American Cancer Society and in 1979 began offering free breast screenings for the Harlem community every Saturday morning.

"I hired a doctor, a nurse, and a clerk and we went out and told people to come up to the seventh-floor clinic on Saturday mornings at nine o'clock," he said. "And we got a big response. People began to come into the clinic, and we began to pick up some early masses, so it looked like it was helping."

The program had been running for perhaps half a year when he ran into his first barrier: the hospital administrators approached Freeman and told him he had to shut it down because he had not obtained proper authorization.

"I had just set it up without getting permission," he recalled. "I had a certain amount of authority being the chairman of surgery, but I didn't have that much."

He was determined to keep the clinic open, though, and so he made an appointment to plead his case with an administrator at the New York City Health and Hospitals Corporation, the government organization that operates the city's public hospitals, including Harlem Hospital. You're trying to do the right thing, the administrator told Freeman, but you aren't doing it the right way. She agreed to help him navigate the bureaucracy and win the corporation's support for the free breast cancer screening clinic.

Several weeks later, she visited him at his office and gave Freeman a coding number he could add to the patients' charts that would entitle them to free care at the weekend clinic. No longer would these women have to wait for hours in an emergency room only to be told they couldn't be seen or be forced to take a day off work to travel downtown and stand in line for a Medicaid card. They would no longer have to spend sleepless nights worrying about the lumps in their breasts and how they might get a doctor to diagnose and treat the problem. And they would no longer be forced to ignore the growing tumors until they became impossible to ignore, by which time it would likely be too late.

"It was like a magic number," Freeman said of the administrator's code. "And from that point on, you've had a free clinic at Harlem Hospital every Saturday."

That new screening system brought about a revolution in outcomes for the women of Harlem who were able to take advantage of it. Between 1964 and 1986, Harlem Hospital treated 606 women for breast cancer, most of them diagnosed before Freeman opened the Saturday clinic starting in 1979. Of these women, 6 percent were diagnosed with stage 0 or stage I cancer, while 49 percent had stage III or IV disease.

Between 1995 and 2000, long after Freeman had established the free clinic, they treated 325 breast cancer patients. They found that 41 percent had stage 0 or stage I cancer, and 21 percent were diagnosed at stage III or IV. Improving the community's access to screening and care appeared to have made a difference.[1]

THE IMPACT OF POVERTY AND RACE ON CANCER TREATMENT

Freeman's most influential work was yet to come, though. In 1988, he was elected president of the American Cancer Society, becoming the first African American to hold the position. As president, he led the organization to focus on questions of race and poverty and their impact on cancer outcomes, an effort that culminated in the publication in 1989 of a study, "Report to the Nation," detailing the inequities and challenges poor Americans faced in obtaining timely, high-quality cancer care.[2]

That report accentuated the difficulty that pioneers like Freeman faced in trying to focus the medical community on a reality that had been well-known, but largely ignored for decades—that they could substantially reduce cancer death rates simply by making screening and treatment more readily available to lower-income and minority communities. To build their case, Freeman and the American Cancer Society worked with the NCI and CDC to collect stories from 250 cancer patients and medical professionals describing the challenges lower-income patients faced in negotiating the healthcare system.

Freeman's interest in the ways poverty and race affected cancer care stemmed from questions he and other experts had started to ask when examining outcomes data. In 1973, his mentors at Howard, White and Leffall, published with colleagues one of the first studies systematically investigating racial differences in cancer mortality in the U.S.[3] (An interesting historical note: the first author named on that study was Ulrich Henschke, chair of radiotherapy at Howard University Medical School and the father of radiologist Claudia Henschke, an influential leader in driving adoption of lung cancer screening.)

Looking at data collected by the NCI, White, Leffall, Henschke, and their colleagues found that between 1950 and 1967 the gap in cancer mortality rates between Black Americans (and Black men, in particular) and white Americans expanded sharply. In 1950, Black Americans had a cancer mortality rate that was 2 percent lower than that for whites; by 1967, Black mortality rates were 18 percent higher than rates for whites.

Freeman had first joined the board of the American Cancer Society in 1978 and chaired a committee focused on cancer issues for minorities. He published studies on the racial differences throughout the 1980s, ultimately concluding that, as he would lay out in the 1989 report, "racial disparities in cancer results are due primarily to differences in economic status."

"I began to raise the question of, 'Why are Black people dying of cancer at a much higher rate'" than whites, Freeman said. "And I was willing to accept whatever the answer was. Because if Black people were dying from cancer at a higher rate because they were Black, then the remedies would be different than if they were dying mainly because they were poor."

Equity was a problem, and it pointed the way to a solution. Or, as U.S. Senator Hubert Humphrey said during the 1971 National Cancer Act hearings, significant reductions in the cancer death rate "calls for no great scientific breakthrough," but simply "a more equitable, just distribution of the resources already available to the more privileged members of our society."

Freeman had a concrete plan for how this "more equitable, just distribution" of cancer care might be achieved.

The American healthcare system is complicated and can be especially daunting for the poor and uninsured, as Freeman's early experience at the Harlem clinic demonstrated. Cancer, too, is complex, and successful early detection and treatment requires regular and sustained engagement with medical providers throughout what are often multistep, multiyear processes.

A basic breast cancer screening program provides a good example. First, patients need to be aware that breast cancer screening is an established and recommended procedure and that it cuts cancer mortality. Next, they need to identify a specific location where they can get a mammogram and determine how they will get there. Also, they need to have health insurance or they may need to apply for Medicaid or some other form of medical assistance.

And that's just the start. Once the patients actually have a mammogram, they may need help understanding what the results mean. If there is an indication they may have a tumor, they may need help scheduling follow-up mammograms if surveillance is recommended, or a biopsy. Patients who turn out to have cancer will enter a new, labyrinthine journey potentially involving years of appointments, imaging studies, and arduous treatments, including surgery, chemotherapy, and radiation, requiring much time off for rehabilitation. The reality behind all these steps is that each one represents a point at which a person, frustrated by the process and its demands, frightened, or unable to shoulder the financial burden, could drop out of the system, allowing the disease to take its lethal course.

OVERCOMING THE NAVIGATION BARRIERS

Technically, many of the women Freeman saw during his first years at Harlem Hospital had access to healthcare. Lower-income women who lacked health insurance could go downtown, enroll in Medicaid, make an appointment at the clinic, and see a doctor. In a practical sense, though, the hurdles they needed to overcome in negotiating those steps severely limited that access. What Freeman realized was that while poor patients no doubt suffered, in many instances, from a lack of insurance, from underfunded facilities in their communities, from shortages of doctors and drugs and equipment, an important challenge they faced was navigating the steps in the healthcare system.

Freeman devised a solution.

"I said to myself, if poor people are running into barriers" accessing healthcare, "then maybe we should help them navigate those barriers," Freeman said. In 1990, to help his patients get through these perilous waters he designed and launched what is known as a patient navigation program, the first one in the U.S. While seemingly straightforward, it was a historic initiative. He hired a pair of local women and trained them to guide Harlem Hospital patients through the breast cancer screening process, followed by treatment, if called for. The navigators provided patients with the attention and follow-up that doctors themselves were typically too busy to offer.

"For example," Freeman said, "the navigator was to be present in the room where the doctor was examining the patient on their first visit, listening to the exchange between the doctor and the patient. And the doctor might finally say, 'Okay, you need to have a biopsy of your breast,' and then the doctor's part is over, because they don't have time to talk much more. But the navigator then took the patient to another room and sat down with the patient and asked questions like, 'Did you understand what the doctor just said to you?' And often the patient did not understand. 'Do you have any problem in getting what the doctor says you need?' And the patient says, 'I don't have health insurance,' or they say, 'I have heart disease and diabetes and the doctor says I need medical clearance,' and they don't know what to do. The navigator will help them get health insurance or help them get medical clearance. Or maybe the patient says, 'I'm afraid, I don't trust the hospital.' The navigator will negotiate that. Whatever the problem was, in that one-on-one between the navigator and patient, it was the navigator's job to solve it and to report to me if they couldn't."

The navigation program first focused on making sure symptomatic women—those coming to the clinic with a lump in their breast or some other complaint—received the treatment they needed. Later, the efforts were expanded to encompass the full breadth of what Freeman called the "cancer continuum," including early detection. The effectiveness of the idea is evident in the fact that hundreds of hospitals and cancer centers around the country have since launched patient navigation programs.

Lynn Butterly is a gastroenterologist and a professor at Dartmouth's Geisel School of Medicine. For the last decade, she has been leading a CDC-funded program, the New Hampshire Colorectal Cancer Screening Program, to improve colorectal cancer screening rates and the quality of testing throughout New Hampshire. Patient navigation plays a central role.

"I personally think navigation is one of the most effective resources we have in medicine," she said.

Follow-up research confirms her observation. Multiple studies have shown that patient navigation programs increase cancer screening rates by an average of 10 percent to 20 percent and rates of follow-up on abnormal findings by 20 percent to 30 percent.

If arranging and undergoing a mammogram is a daunting process for some patients, a colonoscopy can be even worse. To begin with, there's the invasive nature of the procedure, which can discourage some. Then there's the necessary bowel preparation, which takes a full day and can be unpleasant. Patients must go on a clear liquid diet, cutting out all solid food the day before the examination. The afternoon or evening before the procedure they must take medications to fully evacuate their bowels. Topping it off, the colonoscopy itself is a roughly half-hour procedure and typically requires some form of anesthesia. And the patient usually must have an escort to take them home for rest afterward.

In the New Hampshire program run by Butterly, the navigation process consists of a minimum of six areas that are discussed on phone calls with patients. The navigators use those calls to assess and address the potential barriers. They review the bowel prep procedures, confirm appointment schedules, and make sure patients understand their results and any instructions regarding follow-up.

Additionally, navigators ensure that results from the screenings are sent to the patients' primary care providers. (Patients who come to the program without primary care physicians are connected to providers by the navigator.) Translation services are provided when needed, and bowel prep instructions are translated into twenty-six languages spoken among the target population.

In a 2017 paper in *Cancer,* Butterly and her colleagues assessed their system by comparing outcomes from 131 patients who had received navigation support and 75 patients who did not. They found that 96 percent of the patients with the guidance completed their colonoscopies, against 69 percent for the group without the benefit of navigation. The supported patients were also six times as likely to have done adequate bowel prep, a key factor in the procedure's effectiveness. All those supported patients as well as their primary care physicians received the colonoscopy results, compared to 82 percent of the patients who had no assistance.[4]

The program cut down dramatically on patient no-shows, which, Butterly noted, are a major problem in colorectal cancer screening. In the low-income population that the Dartmouth doctors targeted, colonoscopy no-show rates typically range between 25 percent and 40 percent. Among the roughly 2,000 colonoscopies performed during the first six years of Butterly's initiative, the no-show rate was 0.1 percent.

"What happens is, the endoscopy unit has scheduled the room, and you have the equipment and the nurse and the doctor and the tech and the lights and the scope cleaners, all of those costs, but no patient," she said. "So both for the good of the patient and the good of the health system, decreasing no-shows is a major benefit, and is something that patient navigation does extremely well."

That was just one of the many programs proving the concept. In the years after Harlem Hospital launched its pioneering navigator program, similar initiatives popped up around the country. According to an NCI survey, by 2003, roughly 200 U.S. cancer programs were using patient navigation in some form.[5]

In 2005, the federal government passed the Patient Navigator, Outreach, and Chronic Disease Prevention Act, which provided $25 million to fund more patient navigation pilot projects. That same year the NCI issued grants totaling another $25 million in support of nine navigation pilot programs, while the Centers for Medicare & Medicaid Services, CMS, provided its own $25 million in funding to support another nine navigation pilots.

In 2012, the American College of Surgeons required that, starting in 2015, cancer programs seeking accreditation would have to offer some form of patient navigation. There is no single source of authoritative data on the current number of navigators currently at work in the U.S. healthcare system, but membership figures from the Academy of Oncology Nurse & Patient Navigators, a leading professional organization, suggest that the field has seen rapid growth. The academy was launched in 2009 with 100 members; today it has more than 9,000. Thirty years after Freeman came up with the idea, navigation has become an accepted and remarkably effective component of cancer care.

THE COST OF PATIENT NAVIGATION? IT PAYS FOR ITSELF

Even so, consistent funding remains an unfortunate barrier in some locations. While large urban hospitals and cancer centers generally have access to the funding to establish and sustain patient navigation programs, many smaller community health centers do not have the financial wherewithal to maintain them.

Whether they can afford patient navigation often comes down to whether they can win grant funding, said Emmons of Harvard's T.H. Chan School of Public Health. That makes these programs "very unstable," she said. "Usually these grants last two, three years. So a lot of these folks are constantly looking for money."

Often that means healthcare administrators must get creative to obtain the needed financial support.

"We're still struggling, nationally, to fund patient navigation," Butterly said. "Patients love it and medical practitioners love it, but the issue is that funding agencies have limited funding and many competing priorities. On the other hand, there are innovative ways to fund and make navigation sustainable, such as placing the navigator within endoscopy units."

Numerous studies have shown that patient navigation is not just an effective and relatively inexpensive way to improve cancer care, but that it can actually pay for itself. Butterly's team analyzed the cost effectiveness of their navigation initiative and determined that it cut costs by as much as $189 per patient simply by eliminating late cancellations and no-shows.

Similar analyses of other navigation programs have found that, despite the upfront expenses, they ultimately reduce health system spending.[6] A study by Accenture, the consulting firm, found that for every full-time navigator a hospital employs, it adds $150,000 in revenue per year.[7] There is also the more important benefit that the navigators improve patient health and health outcomes.

THE PROBLEMS IN A FEE-FOR-SERVICE HEALTHCARE MODEL

There is an ongoing structural challenge, however—the patient navigator programs do not fit comfortably into the fee-for-service payment models common in the U.S. healthcare system. The fee-for-service approach typically means doctors and hospitals are paid for each discrete patient visit, test, or treatment, one at a time. This model stands in sharp contrast to managed care models, where providers are paid a flat fee for caring for a patient, an approach that generally incentivizes cost-reduction tools such as patient navigation.

In a fee-for-service system, healthcare providers face the puzzle of determining how exactly to bill insurers for patient navigation. Do they bill for each individual phone call or contact with a navigator or for each type of guidance provided? Should charges be increased for patients who require more attention? Should insurers pay different amounts for phone-based or email contact rather than in-person contacts? Should navigation by a qualified nurse be reimbursed at a higher rate than navigation done by a trained employee without that medical qualification?

Integrating patient navigation into fee-for-service healthcare involves answering dozens if not hundreds of questions like those, no matter how exasperating. A whole industry of lawyers, lobbyists, consultants, coding specialists, and technicians has been created to help healthcare providers negotiate, as well as manipulate the statutes, regulations, practices, exemptions, and carve-outs that dictate how medical expenses are paid by insurers.

The current labyrinthine structures in the healthcare financial system present formidable barriers. (It is worth noting that Franz Kafka began his career as an insurance company lawyer.) No matter how successful it has proven in practice, integrating the patient navigation model more comprehensively into the current healthcare system is a daunting task and will require a deep commitment from providers if it is to become a transformative tool.

Sarah Downer is a policy researcher at the Center for Medicare & Medicaid Innovation. She was formerly the associate director of whole person care at Harvard Law School's Center for Health Law & Policy Innovation, where, with her colleague Katie Garfield, she investigated different reimbursement models for patient navigation. She said that while navigation may see some insurer uptake at the margins, she doesn't expect it will make major inroads in the current fee-for-service world. A major issue, she noted, is answering that difficult question of what should be included as a reimbursable navigation service in the first place.

She analogized navigation to chronic care management, a healthcare practice with special characteristics that has carved out a distinct space in fee-for-service systems, including Medicare. As the name suggests, it involves planning and coordination of care for patients with chronic conditions like diabetes or heart disease. Medicare covers this care under its fee-for-service program, and it provides procedural codes that providers can use to bill for treatments and care provided. For instance, there can be coverage for a patient's transit costs going between different healthcare providers or ensuring their compliance with medication regimens.

Defining, in detail, precisely what is and isn't covered by these codes, however, is crushingly difficult in the real world. "At the Medicare-Medicaid conferences I've been to in the past couple of years, there have been entire two-hour-long sessions full of people being like, 'What about this? Does this count? Is this covered? What if this person does this on this day?' The implementation of it is enormously challenging," said Downer. "It's really kind of a mess."

There are some efforts to remedy this situation. Perhaps most notably, in 2024, the Centers for Medicare and Medicaid Services began covering patient navigation for individuals with conditions like cancer that, in the agency's words are "serious, high-risk" and require "development, monitoring, or revision of a disease-specific care plan, and may require frequent adjustment in the medication or treatment regimen, or substantial assistance from a caregiver."[8]

That would unquestionably have a marked impact on cancer care, improving outcomes and reducing costs. But some approaches to instituting patient navigation in the private health insurance business still raise concerns. One issue, said Mandi Pratt-Chapman, a researcher working on health equity and patient navigation at the George Washington University Cancer Center, is that top-tier insurance plans might cover navigation, but lower-priced plans might not—meaning navigation would be unavailable to precisely those we know need it most: the medically underserved.

She suggested that the navigation model might work best if insurers incentivized healthcare providers to use it in their systems by linking reimbursement to measures that produced less-expensive outcomes, as when patients adhere to their recommended courses of treatment under guidance from navigators.

In truth, integrating patient navigation more widely and more thoroughly into our cancer care system would produce a transformation only if it is accompanied by broader coordination of medical treatments with financial, organizational, and bureaucratic structures. That involves reengineering not just the way our system works, but how the players in that system communicate and respond to the broader needs of cancer patients. Cancer patients are generally not aware of how little of that coordination takes place.

"Patients assume that their doctors will collaborate with other doctors and other hospitals, and that there is a system to help them pay their expenses, watch their kids, and even pay for their parking, but there is not," Greg Simon, the president of the Biden Cancer Initiative and a cancer survivor, said at a 2017 National Cancer Policy Forum on Establishing Effective Patient Navigation Programs in Oncology. "We are trying to create the system that patients think we already have."[9]

CHAPTER 7
DEATH BY ZIP CODE

WHEN IT COMES TO BREAST CANCER CARE AND OUTCOMES, there is not one city of Boston but several. To see this with painful clarity one need look no further than the different breast cancer mortality rates by race. Black and white women receive early-detection screening—mammograms—at roughly similar rates. But between 1990 and 2009, Black women in the city went from having a breast cancer mortality rate that was slightly lower than their white counterparts to a rate that was almost 50 percent higher.[1]

The reason for the disparity came after the tests that detected abnormalities. Compared to the white women, research showed that Black women (especially lower-income women on Medicaid) were two to three times as likely to experience delays of more than sixty days in starting treatment for their cancer, a critical lapse that, in the case of lethal, fast-growing tumors, can be the difference between controlling the disease or succumbing to it. In addition, almost half of Black breast cancer patients in Boston changed the hospitals where they received treatment in the first year after their diagnoses, a factor that can disrupt or delay needed care.

In Washington, D.C., there is also evidence of this kind of startling disparity in cancer care. Fewer than 50 percent of the Medicaid patients in the nation's capital with a cancer diagnosis received treatment for their condition, according to figures cited by George Washington University's Mandi Pratt-Chapman in a 2019 presentation on patient navigation.[2] In the capital city's heavily Black Seventh and Eighth Wards, breast cancer mortality is four times the rate for the overall city.

We pointed out in earlier chapters the unsettling racial and economic disparities in cancer screening and care. That inequality leads to worse outcomes and higher healthcare system costs, which affects everyone, poor and privileged. It also means that cancer mortality rates are much higher than they would be if the benefits of good care were shared more evenly and not so heavily influenced by the ethnicity, economic status, or the zip codes of patients.

The factors behind the disparities go well beyond race or class or even purely medical factors. Understanding them, researchers have repeatedly found, requires a much broader consideration of all the interconnected social issues, including the quality of education, quality of housing and safety in the community, food security, and employment opportunities. The policies that could address them, and dramatically improve success in the lagging war on cancer, require a multifaceted attack on all these interrelated social conditions that, we know, influence cancer outcomes. Improving the social determinants of health is a task that goes far beyond the capacity of medical practitioners or hospitals to address. Government must take the lead, from the national down to the local level, but numerous other players also have a role to play. That is a foundational issue in devising the strategies that will achieve real progress in the war on cancer.

In their illuminating book, *The American Health Care Paradox: Why Spending More is Getting Us Less,* Elizabeth H. Bradley and Lauren A. Taylor analyze the power of social determinants in driving public health outcomes. The two researchers, who worked together at Yale University's Global Health Leadership Institute, say that this includes such factors as the "neighborhoods people live in, the food people eat, the air people breathe, the amount of exercise people get, and the jobs people have."[3]

They draw two critical conclusions from this broader perspective. The first is that it helps explain the oft-cited statistic that Americans seem to spend far more than other countries on medical care yet receive worse outcomes. The U.S. has, they note, much lower life expectancies, higher infant mortality rates, lower birth weights, more drug-related deaths, and worse numbers for chronic illnesses such as diabetes, obesity, heart disease, and lung disease. So why, they ask, is the U.S. experiencing these disappointing health metrics despite spending more on medicine?

"Inadequate attention to and investment in services that address the broader determinants of health is the unnamed culprit," Bradley and Taylor write.

The second key point they make is that if spending on important social determinants are factored into the analysis of public health, the U.S. actually comes up short compared to the other countries. European countries devote far more spending per capita on their social safety nets and social support and, as a result, enjoy better public health and health outcomes. The U.S. spends less than 10 percent of GDP on social services, less than half the rates in France, Sweden, Austria, Switzerland, Denmark, and Italy.

Cancer experts have long been aware of the influence of social determinants on patient outcomes. When Senator Hubert Humphrey said fifty years ago that, if all citizens received the same quality of cancer treatment then available at the country's top medical centers, mortality rates would be reduced significantly, he was talking about social determinants of health. When Harold Freeman saw women in Harlem dying of breast cancer because they couldn't take the time to travel downtown and wait in line for a Medicaid card, he was confronting social determinants of health. When the American Cancer Society set its 2035 challenge goal of bringing overall cancer rates down as quickly as they had fallen in the college-educated population, the organization was looking at the problem through the lens of social determinants of health.

The University of Texas's Maria Fernandez struck a similar note when she criticized the notion that "if you build it, they will come," and said that, by itself, access to cancer screening and treatment isn't a panacea. The other impediments need to be addressed to drive early detection forward.

There have been limited efforts to build social factors, and not just medical criteria, into the public healthcare process. For instance, in 2019, the U.S. Preventive Services Task Force announced that it had created a work group to look at how it might designate practices addressing social determinants of health as part of its clinical preventive services, similar to cancer screening or other preventive medical practices.

The task force work group noted that while "evidence is needed that clearly links whether addressing [social determinants] improves health outcomes," it is plausible that better understanding, for instance, of a patient's level of healthcare literacy or "financial . . . or time constraints" could help their doctors tailor more effective care plans, including cancer screening and follow-up treatments.[4]

THE FINANCIAL HURDLES

A significant challenge is persuading hospitals and healthcare systems to invest in things like nurse navigation and screening outreach programs that might not be immediately remunerative but that can help reduce outcome disparities. The medical institutions, not surprisingly, are eager for prompt returns on their investments and it is often not clear that these activities will produce those returns, at least on a desirable scale.

Hospital administrators are often competing with other nearby hospitals for patients, so it makes sense for them to invest in programs that reach underserved people, ensuring that they receive appropriate screenings for illnesses such as colorectal, cervical, or lung cancer. The outreach might bring into the system people it has missed, giving the patients access to things like routine checkups and needed medications.

But what if efforts to increase the community's awareness of screening programs succeed in encouraging people to act, but they go to a competing hospital? And what if, once tested, they also go to a competing hospital for their follow-up and downstream care, which

is usually significantly more profitable? From a business perspective—
and healthcare in the U.S. remains very much a business—the financial
benefits from such cancer screening initiatives are uncertain.

About eight years ago, Len Nichols, a professor of health policy at
George Mason University in Virginia, began to examine this problem.

Then entering his early sixties, Nichols, a leader in health policy
reform and a senior adviser for health policy at the Office of Management and Budget during the Clinton administration, received a grant
from the Robert Wood Johnson Foundation, to examine how payment
reform might be used to help address health equity problems.

After Nichols began researching the question he happened upon
a lecture by Lauren Taylor (coauthor of the book on the paradox of
American healthcare costs), who was then a doctoral student in health
policy at the Harvard Business School. Taylor's research was focused
on social determinants such as income, education level, and neighborhoods and how they affected medical outcomes.

"I was so impressed with her talk, I went up to her afterwards and
I said, 'If you will teach me about social determinants, I will find us
an economic model to incentivize investing in them.' Because it was
obvious after about thirty seconds [of Taylor's talk] that we were un-
derinvesting," Nichols said.

In 2011, Taylor was already working with Elizabeth Bradley on an
initial paper examining why the U.S. seemed to spend more but get less
effective health outcomes than other industrialized countries and they
concluded that devoting more resources to improving social support
such as housing, education, job security, and food security, would create a healthier environment and improve outcomes. The challenge was
building a sustainable funding model involving the many stakeholders.

One solution might be for hospitals to coordinate their efforts and
invest jointly in services such as patient navigators and outreach operations. So in 2018, Nichols and Taylor put forward a plan, which they
described in a paper in the journal *Health Affairs*. They explained how

a funding model developed in the 1970s, called the Vickrey-Clarke-Groves mechanism, could be applied to the challenge.[5]

Traditionally, of course, government fulfills this function, not hospitals, by taxing residents and allocating funds to provide public goods. But in the uneven checkerboard of U.S. government administration, those essential services are not always provided, or provided effectively.

The approach that Nichols and Taylor proposed called for the stakeholders in a system to submit bids to a trusted third-party broker (in their paper, Nichols and Taylor suggest that local social welfare nonprofits could serve as independent brokers) to fund an intervention they collectively desire. The broker then calculates what each stakeholder should pay and what benefit each can expect to see from the targeted intervention.

"There has to be someone to whom each individual stakeholder who could benefit will be willing to reveal their actual true willingness to pay," Nichols said. "That's the key."

Papers on health economics do not usually generate much excitement, and certainly not outside a narrow circle of experts, but in this case the *Health Affairs* article drew an overwhelming reaction.

"We had communities from all over reaching out to us and saying, 'Can we do this here?'" Nichols recalled. It represented one small way that some healthcare providers could collaborate to improve conditions for their disadvantaged patients.

BRINGING A NEW FUNDING MODEL TO POOR COMMUNITIES IN WASHINGTON, D.C.

Kara Blankner, director of programs at the Jane Bancroft Robinson Foundation, a Washington, D.C.-based healthcare nonprofit, was among those drawn to Nichols and Taylor's funding model. Blankner is currently leading the foundation's efforts to use patient navigation to cut cancer mortality among women in some of the city's least affluent communities.

Nichols and Blankner met by chance at a Washington dinner event. During the meal, Nichols introduced her to the funding model he and Taylor presented in their Health Affairs article. That unexpected encounter opened her eyes, Blankner said, to how she might fund some of her objectives. Nichols "was telling me about this economic model, and as soon as he described it, a little alarm bell went off in my head. And I said, 'How do we apply that? How do we take your model and apply it here to cancer navigation?'"

Nichols was, at that time, unfamiliar with the details of patient navigation, so he responded by asking Blankner to explain what it was and how it worked in the cancer field. That launched him on an effort to determine whether the approach he and Taylor had outlined could help Blankner obtain funding.

"You keep a woman alive, you save a lot of money for the society at large," said Nichols. "So there are a lot of stakeholders in improving breast cancer mortality and survival."

The Jane Bancroft Robinson Foundation was formed in 2011 after the merger of D.C.-based Sibley Memorial Hospital with the Johns Hopkins Health System. Endowed with funds released through the merger process, the organization's mission is to help provide healthcare to residents of the city's Seventh and Eighth Wards. Tucked into Washington's southeast corner, these are two of the city's poorest neighborhoods.

Noting the extremely unequal outcomes in cancer care in the wards, the foundation decided that that was an important medical need to focus on. Breast cancer mortality for women in the districts is a multiple of the rate in the rest of the city.

Blankner decided that patient navigators would be one key to achieving the program's goals.

Blankner met with a number of organizers, advocates, and medical professionals from around the city to enlist support and explain the effort to provide patient navigators. At one of those meetings a staff member at the DC Primary Care Association, a healthcare non-profit, warned her that no matter how well-meaning the foundation's efforts were, without reliable, renewable funding for the navigation program it was unlikely to succeed.

It was not long after being given that admonition that Blankner met Nichols at the dinner event and their collaboration was born.

The challenge of providing equitable patient care has other dimensions that health organizations can pursue in collaborations.

Bruce Pyenson, an actuary and expert in the economics of healthcare, cited as one example the impact that good patient follow-up within a screening program can have on reducing "leakage"—the loss of patients from a medical system.

"Often the results from screening are just sent back to primary care and primary care just scratches its head and doesn't really know what to do," Pyenson said. "A more aggressive stance on follow-up, saying, 'Hey, doc, this patient should be followed up at three months, or six months, we'd like to schedule that,' is the kind of thing that is needed. Because otherwise people get lost, or they go outside the system."

This is precisely the type of information a robust patient navigation program can convey within a screening program, a way of aligning good business and good medical practice.

But perhaps the most formidable barrier to building such a comprehensive system and implementing strategies that can deliver excellent outcomes, reducing disparities, is the unusual structure of the American healthcare colossus. Unlike European healthcare systems, which are far more centralized and consistently run by national governments, the American system is largely administered by the private sector and splintered with a range of governmental entities, from the federal government down to states and municipalities, that regulate and oversee care. Cancer care, in particular, is subject to these divided interests.

We have in early detection and treatment of cancer an intricate, multistep process requiring coordination among healthcare professionals. There must be effective outreach to identify and bring at-risk patients into the system, followed by well-run protocols for screening accompanied by timely follow-up and treatment.

There must be methods for keeping track of these patients year after year. There must be sustainable funding models and ways of tracking the dollars as they flow through the system, to show how an investment in one area leads to savings in another, how what might look like cost centers are in fact key to driving profits.

What we need, simply put, is an overarching platform with the ability to grasp the entire process from start to finish, to consider the full scope of the challenge in all its complexities. What we have, though, is a healthcare system seemingly designed to frustrate any such effort— labyrinthine collections of providers, private companies, nonprofits, philanthropies, and government agencies with no comprehensive, inclusive structure encouraging all participants to operate in unison.

The question is whether these pieces can be coordinated to achieve the immensely important goal of reducing cancer mortality, and reducing it equitably. As we'll see in the pages ahead, it can be done.

CHAPTER 8
LAHEY HOSPITAL: A LUNG SCREENING SUCCESS STORY

IN 2009, CLAUDIA HENSCHKE TRAVELED TO THE LAHEY Hospital & Medical Center in Burlington, Massachusetts, to debate one of the hospital's pulmonologists on the pros and cons of what had become her professional mission, expanding use of the lung cancer screening test low-dose computed tomography (LDCT). The visit came during something of a frustrating patch in Henschke's advocacy for this highly effective early-detection technology. She and her professional partner, David Yankelevitz, had lost the argument over whether a randomized controlled trial, the National Lung Screening Trial (NLST), was needed to prove the technology's benefits. They felt that the long trial created an unacceptable delay in bringing the lifesaving test into widespread use.

The trial was well into its seventh year, but most in the medical community had no intention of moving ahead with screening before the results came in. Additionally, a separate lung screening trial, the Dutch-Belgian NELSON study, had been launched in 2003. Those results would also help determine if the LDCT test should be deployed broadly to help reduce deaths from the most lethal of cancers.

For advocates like Henschke, those trials frustrated their efforts to make LDCT a game changer in the efforts to reduce lung cancer mortality. But her visit to the Lahey Hospital & Medical Center began to turn the campaign in her favor, even if just a little.

Andrea McKee is currently the chair of radiation oncology at Lahey and the leader of its lung screening program. At the time of Henschke's visit, McKee was not yet affiliated with the hospital, but her husband, Brady McKee, also a doctor, was. He had joined its staff the year before as a radiologist.

The hospital was hosting a dinner for Henschke following the debate and extended an invitation to Andrea McKee through her husband. Henschke, Andrea McKee recalled, "was like my hero."

"I went to the dinner and, you know, she's just amazing, she's just an incredible pioneer, and I was so struck by what she had to say," Andrea McKee recalled. When she joined Lahey the following year as the head of radiation oncology, she began laying the groundwork for the hospital to widely employ the LDCT lung cancer screening.

McKee had first become interested in lung screening through her work treating early-stage lung cancer patients with a technique called stereotactic body radiation therapy. The treatment involves using intense, precisely targeted bursts of radiation to attack small tumors while sparing surrounding tissue from damage. It is commonly used on patients with early-stage cancers who, usually for reasons unrelated to the disease, are not healthy enough to have surgery to remove their tumors. The results of that therapy were very positive, validating, in her view, efforts to identify and attack the disease as early as possible.

"These patients, who weren't even in good enough shape to have surgery, were living so much longer than the otherwise completely healthy stage IV lung cancer patients I was treating," she said. "And I just became a believer that if we could detect lung cancer early, we could make a big difference in the disease."

McKee all but grew up knowing this was a direction she would take. She said she knew by middle school that she wanted to be a doctor; her motivation took her to a string of elite institutions. She went to college at the University of Pennsylvania then medical school at Columbia followed by a residency at the Memorial Sloan-Kettering Cancer Center.

Her husband, Brady, took a more meandering path to medicine. The couple began dating while undergraduates together at Penn. When

Andrea started at Columbia, Brady went to work in finance, first at a boutique options firm and then at Barclays, the British bank. After eight years, he decided to move to a hedge fund and eventually received an offer—when something unexpected happened: Brady said he realized, more or less out of the blue, that his real dream was to go into medicine.

He enrolled at Hunter College in New York City for his pre-med coursework. A year later, he started medical school at Columbia. When Andrea finished her residency she took a job in New Hampshire, so Brady transferred to Dartmouth. Then, in 2004, he began his residency in radiology at Lahey Hospital & Medical Center and, in 2008, joined the hospital's staff full time.

By the time of Henschke's visit in 2009, Andrea had examined the evidence and was convinced that lung screening could save significant numbers of lives. Brady, on the other hand, was a skeptic.

"I was like, yeah, it's probably all bullshit, there isn't a randomized controlled trial, so it all may just be lead-time bias and overdiagnosis," he said. "It just wasn't a focus for me."

The turning point in his thinking came during a weekly meeting of Lahey's radiology department before Andrea's employment there. The head of radiology was "just kind of a curmudgeonly guy," Brady said. Not, in other words, the sort of doctor likely to impulsively embrace a new or unproven technique.

"We had these conferences every Monday," Brady recalled. "And at one of those conferences, he was just like, it's obvious that we should be doing [lung screening]. Like there's just no question about it. And the combination of hearing that from him and hearing about it from Andrea made me really start to think about it differently."

But the NLST trial was still ongoing. Any steps forward would depend on whether the results supported the effectiveness of the scans.

GETTING FROM A TRIAL
TO A SCREENING SYSTEM

The NCI reported the initial results from the trial in November 2010, showing that LDCT testing cut lung cancer deaths in the large screening group by 20 percent.

"They announced the mortality benefit, and I was like, okay, that's it. We're done. Let's go. Let's do it," Brady said. He put together an email proposing that the hospital launch a mobile lung screening program as soon as possible, a somewhat audacious initiative coming from a doctor so new to the field and the hospital.

"This is me, like a year and a half out of residency telling like the senior people at Lahey that we need to get a truck and we need to start screening people right now," he recalled, laughing. "And they basically said to me, 'Look, we can't do anything, certainly not before [the NLST] is published. But even then, we'll need some national society to issue some sort of guideline statement on it.' And that was it. It was just dropped, essentially, and we just had to wait until the NLST got published."

The full study results were published the following summer in *The New England Journal of Medicine*. It was a milestone. Here, at last, was evidence that lung cancer screening saved lives—the complete protocols and dataset from a 50,000-person randomized controlled trial.

A study is nice, but even a study as extensive as the NLST can only take you so far. Typically, you have to then show that the study's results are generalizable to your particular institution and patient population. This involves a long series of arduous steps.

You have to develop and put in place the training and protocols and personnel required to deliver the intervention. You need quality control processes to make sure your procedures and practitioners are performing well, and you need to prepare plans for taking corrective action when they aren't. You need systems for reaching out to the people you hope will take advantage of the intervention and for keeping track of them and their results. You need to ensure that you can deliver appropriate treatments after those tested become your patients. You need models demonstrating the business case. Then you must gather up all the information and plans and present them to the institution's leadership to convince them the initiative is worthwhile.

This is the challenge of implementation, the challenge Andrea and Brady McKee faced as they tried to take lung cancer screening from a study in an academic journal to a full-fledged clinical program. Passion and data are simply not enough when health is at stake. It's a difficult task in most any case, but particularly so when you're one of the first to take it on. That was the catch in establishing this lung cancer screening program—no one had actually done it yet outside of the trials and academic studies like the one prepared by Henschke and Yankelevitz.

"We didn't really know what to do," Andrea said.

Even so, they pushed forward, assembling one by one the pieces they would need to launch and sustain the program.

In addition to the healthcare it provides locally in Massachusetts, Lahey also provides some medical services to people on the British island territory of Bermuda, which, with a population of around 70,000, doesn't have enough people to support an extensive roster of medical specialists. As part of this relationship, the McKees made a trip to the island shortly after the NLST study was published to give a highly detailed presentation on lung cancer screening.

"As part of that, I had to put this whole business plan together on implementing lung cancer screening in Bermuda," Brady said. "And in order to do that I had to go through the entire NLST and all the tables and basically put together a model on how lung screening would work there. Cost effectiveness, how many cancers they would detect, how many lives saved . . . all based on the NLST results if they were applied to the Bermuda population."

As it turns out, the island has one of the lowest smoking rates in the world, so Brady determined the island would not see much benefit. But the exercise proved useful for preparing the Lahey team back home. A year later, the process took a critical step toward success. The National Comprehensive Cancer Network (NCCN), an authoritative medical body, issued guidelines on lung cancer screening, an essential stamp of approval. That was the push the McKees needed, and by then they were ready to go.

Convincing clinical trial data is great, but the way to persuade the larger medical community that a new intervention will work is to win the endorsement of important professional associations. The average doctor does not have the time to keep up with, or closely scrutinize and evaluate, all the new research affecting the field. Instead, that responsibility is largely handled by professional organizations, which then make recommendations on what new practices doctors should consider adopting.

FINALLY GETTING SCREENING GUIDELINES, AND HITTING THE NEXT HURDLES

In the world of cancer care, the NCCN is respected and influential. It is a collection of thirty-three leading U.S. cancer centers and is one of the leading voices in oncology. The guidelines it prepares and issues are considered by many in the field to be the definitive standards for diagnosing, treating, and managing cancers. Thus the release of its guidelines in 2011 for LDCT screening were critical.

The guidelines dropped online just as Andrea McKee was preparing to give a talk on stereotactic radiation at a conference at the Mount Washington Hotel in Bretton Woods, New Hampshire. Brady saw them and made a quick detour.

"I said, 'I'm going to stay in the hotel room and just read this instead of going to your talk,'" Brady recalled. "And I read it and absolutely everything we needed was in those guidelines. Everything we needed to do the program, everything we needed to justify it, to put a real plan together."

Almost everything. The one piece of the puzzle still missing was a means of paying for the screening system. Even with the guidelines established, plans for reimbursement of LDCT screening by both private and government payers was still several years off.

"It's after the NCCN, we had everything we need, and I was like, how can we do this program?" Brady said. "How can we launch this program at Lahey?"

The answer, he decided, was to provide screening for free. At this initial stage of the process, insurers were still not reimbursing for the test, but it seemed likely they would be in a few years. And free screening might attract patients, at least some of whom would need follow-up treatment, which would bring in revenue. A free program was, in other words, a way to get started quickly and develop expertise while delivering a highly effective service to the community.

"I was driving home from work one day and it just came to me," Brady said. "I started thinking, can we do this for nothing and make it work?"

The McKees and their colleagues had been trying to work out exactly how much they could charge patients for screening and still get enough people through the door to justify the extensive preparation and infrastructure for the program.

"But we realized that we just weren't going to get anyone if we charged anybody anything," Brady said. "We needed to just do it for free."

Predictably, that proposal didn't go over especially well at the hospital. The McKees took it first to several of their fellow radiologists to get their responses.

"They literally just laughed in our faces," Brady said. "They were like, Lahey will never do that."

Nevertheless, the two persisted, approaching the departments that a lung screening program would ultimately affect—pulmonology, oncology, internal medicine—to lobby for support.

They did not always get a warm reception, at least at first. The McKees were convinced of the efficacy of LDCT, and the NLST trial results strengthened their arguments, but they still ran into skepticism about early detection in lung cancer. In one case, Brady recalled approaching a member of the thoracic imaging department about the proposed program—shortly after that doctor had been quoted saying that there was no evidence that lung screening was effective.

"There were a lot of people out there who for decades had been programmed to say, 'Well, there's no real evidence for this, everything is lead-time bias and overdiagnosis and it's all just BS,'" he said. "So we had to show them that it wasn't. And to their credit, when we presented the case, they saw the value."

Like Henschke and Yankelevitz, the McKees are strong critics of the NLST, which they believed was poorly designed and was built to understate the benefits of LDCT screening. But the fact that the trial proved some mortality reduction, despite the limitations of its design, provided some help in making the case for a screening program.

"As weak a study as it was, the fact that it managed to prove a mortality benefit was quite a strong signal that there really was something there," Brady said.

Brady also drew on the years before he became a doctor, when he was an engineer and worked in finance, with their emphasis on heavy data research and analysis, to bolster his explanations for how a program could work and succeed.

"That was the key," Andrea said. "He had been in quantitative analysis. This was his thing."

"If you look at the NLST, there is a lot of information that is only in the tables and not in the text," Brady said. "And so you have to go and recreate the table in a spreadsheet and pull out all that hidden data—the different ratios and all this other stuff. And once you have that, then you have a case you can apply to any other [clinical] situation. But you have to sit down with a spreadsheet and do it. None of it is complicated, but certainly most doctors don't have a lot of experience with that kind of stuff. It's not like they train you to deal with spreadsheets in medical school."

Their persistence, and expertise, finally paid off. The McKees and their colleagues received approval from Lahey's leadership to establish an LDCT lung screening program toward the end of 2011. Now it was time for the real challenge—moving from spreadsheets to actual people in the community.

The difference between an effective screening program and an ineffective or even potentially harmful one comes down to the details, and there was no shortage of details for the Lahey team to iron out.

MAKING SCREENING WORK BY MAKING IT FREE

For starters, the fact that they were offering screening free of charge meant the program had to operate under certain legal restrictions. For instance, it is typically illegal under federal law to advertise medical services being provided for free, which meant the hospital had to come up with alternative ways to reach their targeted populations. For almost two months leading to the program's formal launch, the Lahey doctors held events with local primary care provider groups, laying out the hospital's plans and making the case for screening eligible, at-risk patients.

To gain the support of the primary care doctors, the hospital had to not just make them aware of the screening program, it also had to assure them that the program would not make their jobs harder by adding complex flows of new information. Another challenge was building a system for structuring and sharing the LDCT results so that they could be interpreted consistently at different facilities by different doctors.

Fundamentally, the LDCT test involves trying to detect lesions or nodules in the patient's lungs and then determining whether any such abnormalities are likely to be cancerous, based on criteria like size, shape, and structure. When applying this screening to large populations, involving multiple medical centers, it is critical that the process follows consistent standards.

The process should be reproducible, so that, say, a nodule identified as likely benign in one scan will receive the same evaluation in a future scan (assuming, of course, that it has not grown or changed). The process should be transferable, so that different doctors at different sites will generally reach the same conclusions about any abnormalities (allowing that there will always be borderline cases on which capable doctors may disagree). The process should also be streamlined enough to allow for recording and cataloging the results of hundreds of thousands or even millions of scans, but flexible and nuanced enough to account for the complexity of the disease. All in all, it is a significant medical, logistical, and administrative challenge.

One advantage for the Lahey team was that radiologists had for decades been using just such a system for reading mammograms. Called BI-RADS, for Breast Imaging Reporting and Data System, the program was developed by the American College of Radiology in the 1980s to help standardize the reporting of mammogram results.

The system uses categories numbered 0 through 6 to score the likelihood that a mammogram or other imaging test detects a possible breast cancer. A score of 0 means the test was incomplete. A score of 1 means the test was negative—no lesion was found. A 2 means a lesion was found and it was benign. A 3 means a lesion that is most likely benign. A 4 means a lesion that appears to be a possible cancer. (Within the 4 category some radiologists use the subcategories 4A, 4B, and

4C to indicate increasing levels of suspicion of a malignancy.) A score of 5 means a lesion that is highly likely to be cancer. A 6 means a lesion that has been proven via biopsy to be malignant. Those benchmarks help organize and assimilate the testing results.

Following that precedent, the Lahey radiologists built a system for reading lung LDCTs that they called Lung-RADS.

"If you're going to be screening people every year for decades, you're going to have huge amounts of data, and you are going to have to have a way to assess quality in your program and review the findings," Brady said. "You can't do that without a coding system. That's what had been happening in breast imaging for decades, and that allowed breast imaging to be looked at in a systematic way across the whole country and for programs to sort of compare themselves to standardized benchmarks."

In basing Lung-RADS on the BI-RADS model, the Lahey team also hoped to make the primary care physicians they were approaching more comfortable with the idea.

"We wanted something that was in the language they already understood, and we wanted them to understand that the program would work just like breast imaging, where they aren't expected to get involved in decisions about what to do about a 7 millimeter nodule or an 8 millimeter growing nodule," Andrea said. "Primary care shouldn't be deciding about those situations. That should be coming from the system and the programs."

She continued, "That was part of what we taught them in the campaign. They had very clear instructions as to what their piece of it was. Otherwise, what happens is primary care feels like they are having to deal with this whole thing and it's just too much. They don't have the expertise to deal with it, they aren't comfortable doing it, and they don't even want to engage with it."

Another essential piece of the overall screening infrastructure was building a dedicated database to receive and sort the enormous volumes of data that the system would generate. The Lahey team knew that they ultimately wanted to be screening thousands or even tens of thousands of patients per year, creating a flow of data that no spreadsheet could accommodate. They needed a system that could keep track of the patient contact information, their primary care providers, the radiation doses on the scans they had received, the test findings, any follow-up to those findings and how they were resolved, and when the patients were due for their next scans. The team went to work constructing that database.

Another step involved additional training for the radiologists who would conduct and evaluate the LDCT scans. They were typically well-versed in evaluating incidental lung nodules that were detected when a patient received a CT scan for some other purpose unrelated to lung screening—to check for injuries, for instance, after an auto accident. Interpreting a scan done explicitly for screening purposes requires somewhat different expertise, though, and thus some additional instruction is called for. To account for that, the Lahey team set up an internal training and certification program to make sure the doctors reading the LDCT screenings had the necessary capabilities.

The dozens of large and small decisions and accommodations that went into that marathon to establish the hospital's program might have seemed to prove the nagging possibility that the LDCT skeptics were right after all. Maybe it is too heavy a lift with too many opportunities for costly failure.

But there was a larger truth behind the Lahey effort: it ultimately demonstrated, those involved believed, just how much room there was to improve upon the modest results of the NLST trial. It was clear to many of those involved that, once the team had navigated all those steps and built their system, the 20 percent mortality benefit from the trial might well be a floor rather than a ceiling.

Lahey Hospital & Medical Center launched its LDCT early-detection lung screening program in January 2012. Since then, it has carried out nearly 27,000 examinations, screening more than 7,700 patients. Over that time, the hospital has seen a remarkable stage shift in the lung cancers it treats, indicating the effectiveness of its program. In 2011, it saw seventy-eight patients with stage I disease and sixty-seven with stage IV disease—roughly equivalent numbers. By 2021, the number of stage I patients had nearly doubled to 137, while the number of stage IV patients had fallen by more than 30 percent, to forty-four. Perhaps most important, Lahey screens about 60 percent of its eligible population, compared with the roughly 4.5 percent level nationwide.

"We didn't get caught up with, oh my gosh can we do this, can this be done?" Andrea McKee said. "We believed from the get-go that this could be done and could be done well. Like any complex problem, you have to look at the barriers and you have to develop systems to address them. And that was what we did."

Postscript: Tragically, Brady McKee died in an accident in 2022. We offer our deepest condolences to Andrea and his family. His death is a tremendous loss to all who knew him and to the field of cancer screening.

CHAPTER 9

OVERCOMING UNEQUAL TREATMENT IN EARLY-DETECTION PROGRAMS

THE EFFORT TO REDUCE CANCER DEATHS IS LARGELY A numbers game. We define real progress not by ones and twos, not by positive stories of miraculous treatments saving a few lives, but by how we can reduce the mortality rates among very large populations— never forgetting that each digit represents thousands of husbands and wives, parents and children, friends, neighbors, rich and poor, ordinary people hoping they can navigate life without the threat of a cancer diagnosis interrupting it all.

Innovative medical care and research are essential to that effort. Dedicated healthcare professionals are irreplaceable elements. The effort is so large that focused government support and funding must be integral to any strategies to achieve real results at scale. Still, a major challenge lies in our need to devise and deploy highly effective systems that can harness the specialists, administrators, insurers, and funders to manage entire populations in diverse locations and involving many income levels.

That reality may not have the imaginative sparkle of "Eureka!" medical breakthroughs that transform defeat into success, but mastery over the vast range of details in those systems for diagnosing and treating the disease, the skilled management needed to build and maintain progress, is its own kind of heroism. The National Committee for Quality Assurance is little known outside healthcare circles, but it is arguably one of the more influential bodies in medicine. A nonprofit based in Washington, D.C., the committee was formed thirty years ago to create standards for evaluating the quality of managed care plans like health maintenance organizations (HMOs) or pre-ferred provider organizations (PPOs).

At the time it was created, managed care was a fast-growing part of the health insurance landscape (it has since exploded in size, becoming the main route by which healthcare is provided in the U.S.), and different plans were looking for ways to distinguish themselves from competitors. The benefits covered by many plans were roughly the same, as were costs and provider networks. As a result, metrics that distinguished the quality of care became a primary means of differentiating the managed care programs and enhancing their marketing.

The committee thus had to define quality and construct meaningful metrics. Generally speaking, quality in the provider context has come to mean that the care patients receive has proved to lead to improved health outcomes for large populations, supported by statistical evidence, and that the providers deliver this care comprehensively and consistently. In other words, high-quality care means that a large percentage of a managed care plan's patients are up to date with the recommended colorectal cancer screenings, for example. Lower quality might mean that relatively few patients receive timely screenings or that doctors use outdated or unproven screening approaches.

The quality assurance committee has built a performance measurement known as the Health Plan Employer Data and Information Set, or HEDIS, which tracks more than ninety metrics to score performance. The committee says that 191 million people, or more than half the country, are enrolled in plans that employ the HEDIS system for monitoring quality standards. Some Medicare insurance plans and some state Medicaid plans are required to submit HEDIS data annually to help track their quality. Participation is voluntary for private insurers but many use it, as it provides them with an independent assessment of plan effectiveness.

This means that scoring well is a priority, and thus insurers build their plans with incentives to increase the metrics calculated by HEDIS. For instance, they can offer doctors incentives, such as bonuses, for hitting certain thresholds for patient care. A medical practice might receive a bonus payment if 80 percent of its female patients aged 50 to 74 receive an annual mammogram, a HEDIS metric. Get that percentage up to 90 percent and the bonus might rise.

When applied to large populations, the incentives clearly work. Breast cancer screening and colorectal cancer screening are both tracked under the HEDIS guidelines. Adoption rates for the two are just below 80 percent and 70 percent, respectively. Lung cancer screening, however, is not in the HEDIS guidelines. This is among the reasons that less than 10 percent of the eligible population is being screened.

Every year the committee puts out a summary report scoring the different plans it evaluates along three axes—patient experience, prevention, and treatment. Each plan is rated in these categories on a scale of 1 to 5, with 1 being the worst score and 5 the best. For early-detection cancer screening, the relevant category is prevention. In the 2019–2020 ratings, four private insurance plans received a 5 for prevention and all four were, interestingly, from the managed care organization Kaiser Permanente.[1]

There is an important lesson in that data. Beginning with its origins as a health plan developed to cover San Francisco Bay Area shipyard workers during World War II, Kaiser has always made preventive care a priority. In the 1950s, the company began exploring the use of what medical director Morris Collen termed "multiphasic screening," the use of regular testing of individual members even before they show any symptoms of health problems—essentially a form of early detection.[2] In the 1980s, a team led by a Kaiser researcher, Joe Selby, used data collected from sigmoidoscopies of patients in the multiphasic screening program to advance the case for colorectal cancer screening. [3]

This approach, in other words, is baked into the company's business model. Kaiser's founding physician, Sidney Garfield, started his career in medicine by providing care to some 5,000 workers who were building an aqueduct in California's Mojave Desert to bring water from the Colorado River to Los Angeles. He built a twelve-bed hospital near the worksite and began seeing patients on the usual fee-for-service basis. But insurers nearly bankrupted his practice with slow payments and denial of payments for some procedures.

So he adopted a different financial approach, a prepayment model. The workers paid him a flat fee upfront and in return they received any medical care they needed. It was a precursor, essentially, of what is now called managed care.[4]

As Garfield quickly came to see, preventive medicine was key to making his system work. While fee-for-service doctors have an incentive to do as many procedures as possible, a managed care model pushes them in the opposite direction. Patients pay the same amount regardless of how much medical care they receive, so medical practices earn more by reducing the amount of treatment they need to provide. The healthier their members, the higher their earnings. And the sooner doctors can identify and treat illnesses the lower their costs. It's a model that meshes well with an emphasis on early detection.

ELIMINATING RACIAL DISPARITIES IN CANCER OUTCOMES

Several years ago, researchers from Stanford and the University of California, San Francisco, looked at racial and ethnic disparities in colorectal cancer mortality across some California healthcare systems. The results were fairly predictable. As the American Cancer Society showed in its study of contrasting colorectal cancer outcomes for Black and white patients, the introduction of widespread screening had actually widened racial disparities around colorectal cancer, not narrowed them, and this finding held true for the systems that the researchers investigated, with one exception. In one system the researchers found no differences in outcomes across racial or ethnic groups.[5]

They didn't name the system in the paper, but it was identified in an accompanying editorial as Kaiser Permanente.[6]

So how did Kaiser do it? To hear Kim Rhoads, one of the paper's authors and an associate professor of epidemiology and biostatistics at the University of California, San Francisco, describe it, the answer would seem to be "almost without meaning to."

"I don't think they deliberately set out to address disparities," Rhoads said. Rather, it was simply a result that followed naturally from some of the organization's practices and processes.

First, of course, is its historical emphasis on prevention and early detection. Kaiser's screening rates for breast, cervical, and colorectal cancer are all well above the national averages.

There is also the highly standardized way Kaiser provides medical care. Some have criticized this model as sterile and robotic and at times unable to properly treat particularly complex cases that require creative or innovative care. But it does appear to perform well overall. It is useful to look back for a moment at the idea of evidence-based medicine, the notion that, instead of being guided by tradition or conventional wisdom or the preferences and experience of individual providers, medicine should be based on a set of rigorously validated and consistently applied practices. That approach is central to Kaiser's medical care.

Having done a rotation at Kaiser during her own surgical residency at UCSF, Rhoads is familiar with the system.

"It's very routinized, the way they provide care," she said. "There's kind of a recipe for how you do what you do, and there's not a lot of choice. I think this is the secret behind [the system's results in eliminating disparities]. If you take 100 patients and you treat them all the same, you are going to get a bell-shaped curve where 95 percent do well, 2.5 percent are going to do super, and another 2.5 percent are going to do really badly."

Compare this to how medicine is often practiced outside of managed care systems. Doctors usually have more discretion in screening for cancer, follow-up, and treatment, and thus practices can vary widely from doctor to doctor.

"You're not going to get a bell-shaped curve in a system like that, if you can even call it a system," Rhoads said. However, that is still how much of American healthcare is conducted.

Integration of medical services is also key to the way Kaiser delivers care. Under his vision, Garfield brought into close coordination the many players involved in each patient's care, "bringing," as he said, "the doctors' offices, laboratory, x-ray, and hospital . . . all together under one roof."[7]

"Because it's an integrated system, any time you make contact with the system, they have access to what you're due for," said Harvard behavioral scientist Karen Emmons, who once headed Kaiser's Foundation Research Institute. "If you call up and say, 'I just stubbed my toe really hard, and I think it might be broken,' the appointment person will say, 'Absolutely, we'll get you in for a visit, and by the way, I notice that you're due for your colon cancer screening.' It's about giving care to the whole person as opposed to giving [separate] care to the colon and the toe and the this and that. It's really an excellent model."

The successes of that managed care model present both an opportunity as well as a troubling indication of the poor job the medical system is doing overall in preventive care and early-detection screening. What is the best approach to help the population that has no health insurance, or that is in plans that do not prioritize prevention? Is there any hope of recreating the success of a tightly coordinated system across the atomized enterprises and institutions and arrangements that constitute so much of the country's healthcare landscape?

There might be.

LEARNING FROM DELAWARE

In 2001, the age-adjusted mortality rate for colorectal cancer in the state of Delaware was 20.4 out of every 100,000 residents.[8] That put it slightly above the overall U.S. rate of 20.2 per 100,000.[9] For white residents, the state's colorectal cancer mortality rate was 19.9 out of 100,000 while for Black residents it was significantly worse, 31.2 out of 100,000[10]—in line with the highly unbalanced overall U.S. rates of 19.9 per 100,000 for whites and 28.2 for Blacks.

But in 2009, the story had dramatically improved. Colorectal cancer mortality in Delaware had fallen to around 16 deaths per 100,000 population that year. In and of itself this was not a unique achievement. The U.S. rate had dropped by roughly the same amount, to 15.8 per 100,000. But what was striking was this: Delaware's Black mortality rate was only 18 per 100,000, well below the national rate of 22.4 per 100,000 and almost as low as the 16.9 rate for white Delaware residents. In less than a decade, the state had essentially closed the Black-white gap in colorectal cancer outcomes. How did the state do it?

Throughout the 1990s, Delaware typically ranked among the worst states in cancer death rates. Toward the end of the decade, this stain on the state's healthcare system drew the interest of the state's largest newspaper, the Wilmington-based *News Journal,* which ran a series of stories describing the unusually high number of cancer deaths.

The cancer problem also attracted the attention of the incoming governor, Ruth Ann Minner, whose husband had died of lung cancer nine years earlier. She prioritized improving healthcare and, among other steps, battled the business community to start one of the country's first bans on smoking in public spaces. Her key initiative when she took office in 2001 was assembling a team of experts to formulate an overarching cancer action plan to address the dismal statistics. This was not the first such effort by the state to develop a plan, but this time officials would act, the governor vowed.

"There were a couple other [plans] that had been developed that were just collecting dust on a shelf," said Stephen Grubbs, an oncologist and a member of Minner's cancer study group.

As its mortality rates made clear, Delaware's cancer problem was deep. But, as Grubbs explained, the aim was not to take it all on at once. The strategy was to begin by identifying a smaller, discrete piece of the challenge that the state would have a better chance of improving. The cancer group could then use what it learned from that effort to develop a broader strategy for tackling the larger health issues. When the group surveyed the data to identify a good focus for the initial cancer reduction project, they landed on colorectal cancer as an obvious opportunity. The means for accomplishing their objective was going to be early detection.

"Our screening rates in Delaware for breast cancer were good, for cervical cancer they were good, but for colorectal cancer, like everybody in the early 2000s, they were terrible," Grubbs said.

As a practicing oncologist, Grubbs had a close-up perspective on the consequences of those low screening rates.

"It had certainly left an impact on me, seeing relatively young people dying of colorectal cancer who shouldn't have," he recalled. "It was like, wait a minute. What the hell is going on here?"

There's one case in particular that still troubles Grubbs when he reflects on those poor screening rates and the devastating—and unnecessary—impact they had on some families.

"The sentinel event for me was ... a consultation in the hospital one evening in Wilmington, and I had a vibrant African American woman in her early fifties with advanced colon cancer and a wonderful family, and I just looked at it, and I thought, this should never happen," he said. "It should just never happen. We have the tools to prevent this. That was maybe twenty-five, thirty years ago, and it has stayed with me ever since."

In 2001, Governor Minner signed the resolution establishing the Delaware Advisory Council on Cancer Incidence and Mortality. Two years later, that morphed into the Delaware Cancer Consortium, which focused on the strategy of advancing early-detection screening for colorectal cancer.

Minutes from the group's meetings going back to 2003 are posted on the Delaware Cancer Consortium website and they reveal an important reality—the success of these public health initiatives rests heavily on the seemingly mundane logistical and organizational details that actually bring the program into contact with patients and healthcare providers. There is precious little high-minded talk of cutting-edge science or game-changing wonder drugs. Instead, the minutes show how the meetings focused on cellphone budgets, car mileage allowances for care coordinators, the preparation of PowerPoints for presenting plans to potential hospital partners, and updates on media strategies for reaching at-risk patients in underserved communities. Public information was a critical element in the public health initiative.

"We took the literature at the time and looked at all the aspects of how you get effective screening," Grubbs said. "Not just how do you do it, but how do you mobilize people, how do you navigate, and then what happens after you make a diagnosis."

Like Brady McKee, Grubbs, who for more than a decade chaired the consortium's Early Detection and Prevention Subcommittee, trained as an engineer before becoming a doctor. It was a background that served him well when it came to the group's more pragmatic organizational work.

"It was really a systems engineering problem, using medical things we all knew about and then handing off to a treatment program," he said. "Putting all the known [interventions] together that had evidence, from soup to nuts, and then getting people through it."

And, of course, since the initiative required sustained funding, it also had a political dimension. The organization needed allocations of public funding both for its own operations and to cover the colorectal screen-ing and treatment for residents who lacked insurance or money to cover the costs.

"If we're going to go out there and screen those who are disadvantaged, which is really where the [mortality] gap was, what were we going to do when we find a cancer?" Grubbs said. "It's not going to be effective unless we have a treatment program. That was the second key part of this."

The state stepped up to make that piece work, too. To strengthen support for lower-income cancer patients, Delaware Health and Social Services adopted regulations in 2004 that called for the state to pay for one year of cancer treatment for any uninsured resident with a household income less than 650 percent of the Federal Poverty Level. It has since been extended to two years.

"We did a back of the envelope calculation on how many cancer [patients] we thought were uninsured and what would be the cost to the state to pay for a year's worth of cancer treatment for all of the uninsured," Grubbs said. "We came up with about $4 million, and the legislature bought that. So we built an effective screening program, and then we had a cancer treatment program to hand off to for those who were diagnosed. So now you had the entire equation."

MAKING "SCREENING FOR LIFE" A REALITY

The initiative worked like this: The consortium developed marketing campaigns and relationships with local community organizations to reach their targeted patient groups—underscoring the critical role that mass media and social media campaigns must play in these programs. At the same time, it provided funding for each of the state's five major hospitals to hire nurse navigators to take patients through every step from the outreach efforts through the colorectal cancer screening process and on to any follow-up that was needed. The state covered the cost of screening for uninsured patients through what it called its Screening for Life program, and free coverage was available for qualified patients for the two years of treatment.

The outreach and patient navigators brought the patients. The state coverage attracted and supported the work of the doctors and the hospitals. Screening and care for uninsured patients was reimbursed at the same rates provided by Medicare, which pays more generously than most state-administered insurance programs. That helped alleviate the free-rider problem and other concerns that have limited some hospitals' investments in cancer screening programs.

"Right off the bat, what [providers] were going to be reimbursed . . . was attractive," Grubbs said. "So we could say, 'Here it is, folks, we're going to get you patients, you're going to be reimbursed properly, and we want this to work.'"

Between 2002 and 2009, the state's colorectal cancer screening rates rose from 57 percent to 74 percent, with screening rates for Black residents rising from 48 percent to 74 percent. By 2009, Delaware had also nearly eliminated its Black-white mortality gap for colorectal cancer. Not only that, it had done the job essentially for free. By detecting more colorectal cancers in the early stages, the state saved an estimated $8.5 million a year. That has been more than enough to cover not only the $1 million a year cost of the screening program itself, but also the $6 million per year the program pays in treatment costs for uninsured cancer patients.

"There's a message there," Grubbs said. "If you do medicine properly, use the science, and get it done properly, you will have a more effective, more efficient, healthcare system. So not only do you save lives, but you save dollars."

Another important element in the continuing success of the program is that the state has not wavered in its support. The early-detection initiative was established by a Democratic governor and Democrats have led Delaware ever since (holding the governorship and senate since 1993 and the governorship, senate, and house since 2008), so there has been some continuity in political leadership.

Also, as Grubbs pointed out, several of the politicians originally involved in launching the project have continued their involvement, most notably the current governor, John Carney. He was the lieutenant governor under Minner and he played an important role in supporting the program in its early days. When the group that ran the program published a paper in 2013 in *The Journal of Clinical Oncology* describing the initiative, Carney, who was at that time the state's U.S. representative, was listed as the third author.

"That makes him the only sitting congressman that I know of who was also an author in *The Journal of Clinical Oncology*," Grubbs said.

But the most important reason that the early-detection program has enjoyed continued support from the state is that it has delivered impressive results, saving thousands from avoidable early deaths, and it delivered those benefits relatively quickly.

"I told the legislators, 'Listen, changing the course of cancer takes a long time, but here's an opportunity where I believe you'll see a change in a very short period, and as a legislator you can take credit for it,'" Grubbs said. "And they all have, and appropriately so.

"We were not going to launch a program without collecting data," he said. "Every year when the finance committee comes together in the legislature, we present them data on the outcomes of the money spent on these programs. And the challenge I like to give them is, show me a program in Delaware where you can show results like these for the dollars you've spent."

The committee has now used the same model to expand its work into reductions of other cancers, with programs to promote screening for cervical, breast, prostate, and lung cancer. Since launching the lung cancer program in 2015, the state has brought LDCT screening to roughly 20 percent of its eligible population.[11] While that might not sound like much, it's about double the rate nationwide.

The overall effectiveness of the program has been dramatic. When Minner took office, Delaware ranked second-to-worst—forty-ninth—in cancer mortality. In 2020 the state was thirty-second, middle of the pack, according to the CDC.[12] And while "middle of the pack" may not be the most striking boast, that seventeen-spot improvement represents many early deaths prevented. And it is important to note that they were saved not by a marvelous new technology or a groundbreaking drug, but by using screening technology already available, implementing it in a smart, coordinated, comprehensive, and consistent manner.

Delaware was, in a way, well suited for a trial run of a statewide cancer screening program. With a population of just under a million people, it is small enough to be manageable, but it still has all the complexities that challenge any large-scale public health project—a disparate population, political and budgetary challenges, dispersed, competing healthcare networks, a mix of public and private insurance regimes. Grubbs suggested that the consortium could potentially serve as a model that larger states could emulate.

"The question is, how do you take an incubator in healthcare that a state like Delaware can be—where you have all the government apparatus in place, all the healthcare systems in place, and yet is manageable enough to actually move the needle—how do you take what you learned there and move it to a larger state and deploy it?" he asked.

Even with its overall progress, Delaware has grappled with some setbacks. Cancer is a complex disease and the process of trying to manage it with public health initiatives rarely moves in a straight line. After a decade of initial declines, the state's colorectal cancer incidence and mortality numbers began ticking back up. Incidence hit 35.4 cases per 100,000 residents in 2012. By 2016, that figure had risen to 39.3 cases. Mortality was 13.1 per 100,000 in 2011. In 2017 it was 13.8.[13] But both measures resumed their downward trends in 2018. The state has yet to hit its goal of having 80 percent of residents current with colorectal cancer screening; as of 2020, it was at 77 percent.[14]

The uneven progress is for several reasons. The 2008 financial crisis and subsequent recession wreaked havoc with state budgets, including Delaware's. In the aftermath of the crisis, the state cut the cancer consortium's funding, including its marketing budget. The state also reduced subsidies for nurse navigation, a critical element in the initial success. Both of those factors likely contributed to the decline in screening rates.

Another factor was shifts in insurance coverage for many patients, which appears to have reduced the amount of information patients were provided about the benefits of early detection.

When the Affordable Care Act, or ACA, commonly called Obama-care, came into effect in 2014, it reduced the ranks of the uninsured by expanding Medicaid coverage and providing subsidized private coverage through government-run exchanges. As a result, many people previously covered by Delaware's Screening for Life program used Medicaid or the exchange-based insurance to pay for screenings. In fact, by 2016, around two-thirds of patients previously covered by Screening for Life were using insurance provided through the ACA.

It turned out this was a mixed blessing. The Screening for Life program placed great emphasis on proactively educating and recruiting patients for cancer screenings. That, however, was often not provided under the Medicaid or exchange-based plans. That difference in approach appears to have affected the state's screening and mortality rates.

In addition, many of the ACA plans had high deductibles, which meant patients could face significant out-of-pocket costs for expensive treatments. This wasn't much of an issue for the early-detection screening, because federal law mandates that services recommended by the government's Preventive Services Task Force must be covered without a copay or cost-sharing. The concern, Grubbs noted, was that those high deductibles could deter some patients from getting needed follow-up testing and treatment.

"There are these little pitfalls you run into along the way," he said, "all these little details that you don't think about until you get into it."

Even a successful effort, in other words—something like the Lahey lung screening program or Harold Freeman's navigation project or Maria Fernandez's outreach along the Texas-Mexico border—is always a work in progress. Effective screening depends on too many small but essential—and endlessly changing—variables to ever consider the job done. But the rewards are, unquestionably, substantial. Pay attention to the details, provide sustained funding, and ensure proper follow-up and thousands of deaths will be prevented, year after year.

CHAPTER 10
ON THE CUSP OF A REVOLUTION

WE HAVE EXPLORED THE CURRENT LANDSCAPE OF CANCER early detection, surveying the technologies available and advocating for how they should be used to substantially advance and, finally, start to win the war on cancer. It is within our reach. There are many extremely promising opportunities to improve cancer screening rates for the population groups most at risk, saving what would be many thousands of lives a year—particularly by increasing screening for lung cancer. At the same time, these approaches give us the opportunity to narrow and eventually eliminate the unacceptable disparities in screening and treatment between whites and other ethnic and racial groups and between residents of urban versus rural areas.

The gains from these policy changes would be real, the numbers meaningful, even historical in their significance. But this is just the first part of the transformative opportunity before us. As we will describe, we stand on the threshold of a wave of early-detection breakthroughs.

The real revolutionary transformation begins with an understanding of two critical limitations in our early-detection arsenal. First, the tests—currently for five common forms of cancer—each screen for just a single type of cancer when we must contend with the reality that there are hundreds of different types of cancer that can strike. Second, there simply are no good screening tests yet for the majority of cancers. The cancer types we have discussed—lung, breast, prostate, colorectal, and cervical—are responsible for about 45 percent of cancer deaths in the U.S. annually; tragically, only a small fraction of those lethal cancers were initially detected through screening, which frequently means the patients became aware of the malignancies only after symptoms surfaced, which is often in the later stages. Those figures make clear the need both to sharply increase screening rates as well as to find effective early-detection tests for the cancers that elude us.

Bert Vogelstein, the Johns Hopkins researcher and cancer pioneer, has advocated that we flip the highly unsatisfactory early screening figures, reaching a level in five to ten years in which as many as 75 percent of cancers are detected by early screening tests, meaning at the very early, highly treatable stages, and only 25 percent or so are detected after symptoms emerge.[1]

Finally, that goal appears within sight.

A number of companies have developed or are developing tests that can identify a wide range of cancers in their early stages by detecting aberrant bits of genetic material that these malignancies shed, or turn loose, into the bloodstream. Importantly, these tests are able to pick up not only cancers like lung, breast, and prostate malignancies, which we are already able to detect, but dozens of other cancers—perhaps more than fifty—that the conventional early-detection technologies miss.

Stephen Ezell, in an article for the Information Technology and Innovation Foundation, argued that "it is simply not feasible to spend decades in developing and testing new screening approaches for every single individual cancer." He thus urges that more effort be put into developing the nascent tests that hold the promise of testing for multiple cancers at once. "Multicancer early-detection approaches could make significant contributions to increasing the cancer detection rate in the general population, ideally at earlier stages when, for most cancers, treatment options and potential prognoses are far better," he wrote.[2]

To give one example of how these new tests and wider use of screening could affect mortality rates, women who are initially diagnosed with epithelial ovarian cancer at its latest stages have a five-year survival rate of about 30 percent, while more than 90 percent of women diagnosed at the earliest stages survive at least five years.[3]

In a calculation of the impact of better screening rates, researchers determined that if 33 percent of all metastatic cancers were diagnosed at stage III, rather than stage IV, 33 percent at stage II, and another 33 percent at stage I, there would be 81 fewer deaths per 100,000, a significant 24 percent reduction in cancer deaths, or nearly 150,000 every year.[4]

Some of the advanced early-detection tests rely on a sophisticated understanding that scientists have developed of cancer's once-mysterious genetic and biochemical processes. Using technologies like DNA sequencing, researchers can better identify abnormal, and dangerous, cells or genomes, understand how they became corrupted, and identify where in the body they originated.

That new science has been supplemented with the development of computer-driven bioinformatic techniques that employ machine learning and artificial intelligence for a deeper analysis of the vast amounts of data already being collected through blood draws and other sources. Artificial intelligence, AI, is, in theory, well suited to taking the masses of data produced from screening large numbers of people and discerning patterns—and, importantly, deviations from healthy patterns—that will help doctors identify and target malignancies for early treatment. AI may also, in some cases, help predict which patients are at greater risk and should be subjected to more intensive screening.

Detecting cancers by observing changes in certain cells or cellular processes in our bodies is not by itself a new idea. That's how PSA testing works, with rising PSA levels indicative of potentially threatening abnormalities. What is new is that scientists can now look at the behavior of many different molecules and cells, in thousands of different patients, compare the data and use that information to identify previously unknown patterns that are markers for disease.

By relying not just on tests of a single marker or single type of cancer, as is done in a traditional test like PSA or the Pap smear, but rather by being able to spot multiple disease markers, doctors will possess much more powerful and comprehensive early-detection tools.

SEARCHING FOR ANSWERS IN BLOOD SAMPLES

The promise of these new technologies represents a paradigm shift in the war on cancer. Billions of dollars have started to flow into innovative start-ups that are pioneers in developing new classes of blood-based screening tests. Savvy entrepreneurs like Jeff Bezos and Bill Gates have made investments in companies that are aiming to provide a wave of cancer screening breakthroughs. The pioneers include GRAIL and Thrive Earlier Detection (acquired in 2020 by Exact Sciences).

"The blood is a very rich source of information about cancers in the body, because tumors shed a lot of information into the bloodstream, including cells, circulating tumor DNA, and other molecules that we can collect and analyze," Catherine Marinac, a member of the Faculty of Medicine at the Dana-Farber Cancer Institute, says in the Information Technology and Innovation Foundation article.

One of the most hopeful aspects of these blood-based tests is the prospect that a single draw from patients will allow doctors to detect dozens of cancers at such an early stage that they are far more likely to be cured or halted in their progress. GRAIL's Galleri test can also, it appears, identify with great accuracy where the cancers originated in the body, improving the treatment prospects.

If the tests work as hoped they may, over time, reduce costs and simplify the screening process. Comprehensive cancer screening may become part of the annual checkup, a matter of routine.

Barbara McAneny, an oncologist and former president of the American Medical Association, praised the new early-detection technologies as "amazing science" and a "remarkable advance." But she also warned that implementing the tests as routine elements of a primary physician's annual work would require significant preparation and improvements in physician training and support to avoid doctors being overwhelmed by the details of new screening tools.

"We need algorithms set up so that we make it easy for screening to occur so that both doctors and patients understand that you can go to your primary care doctor, you get a consultation, you learn what you are at risk for, and you set up a plan," she said.

The idea of identifying malignancies by detecting tiny fragments of DNA that have been shed from the abnormal cells into a person's bloodstream (called cell-free DNA, or cfDNA) isn't new. Scientists demonstrated that as far back as 1948, several years even before James Watson, Francis Crick, Rosalind Franklin, and Maurice Wilkins helped discover the double helix structure of DNA.

Three decades after that, researchers showed that some cancer patients had elevated levels of cell-free DNA in their blood serum. In the late 1980s, scientists at the University of Geneva found that a portion of this cfDNA came from tumor cells.

In 1991, a team at Johns Hopkins University found that urine from bladder cancer patients contained DNA with mutations specific to their tumors. Three years later, Dartmouth University scientists showed they could detect mutated forms of the gene KRAS, which are present in almost 15 percent of cancers, in the blood of pancreatic cancer patients. Those insights are among the scientific building blocks of this new generation of screening technologies.

STUMBLING ON A CANCER BIOMARKER

Interestingly, one of the first concrete examples of the technique's feasibility came from a genetic testing technique—called noninvasive prenatal testing, or NIPT—unrelated to oncology.

NIPT uses sequencing of fetal DNA floating free in the mother's bloodstream to test for genetic abnormalities like Edwards Syndrome or trisomy 21 (Down Syndrome). Introduced for clinical use in 2011, the technique has seen rapid adoption, since it offers a safe and convenient alternative to amniocentesis, which requires inserting a long needle through the abdominal wall into the mother's uterus and extracting amniotic fluid.

In 2013, doctors at the University of North Carolina received NIPT results for one of their patients indicating that the fetus had Down Syndrome. When they followed up the NIPT result with amniocentesis, though, they detected no genetic abnormalities. They performed NIPT again several weeks later and again received a result indicating Down Syndrome. An ultrasound showed an apparently normal fetus, however, with subsequent ultrasounds also showing normal development. Ultimately, the baby was born at term, healthy and with no complications or Down Syndrome.

In the weeks after delivery, though, the mother developed pain in her pelvis. Her doctors did imaging and found tumors in her pelvis and stomach that they determined were from a neuroendocrine cancer that had metastasized. And then they made an unexpected discovery: when they analyzed biopsies of these tumors, they found the same genetic abnormalities that the NIPT had detected. The abnormal DNA, in other words, hadn't come from the fetus, it had come from the mother's undiagnosed tumors. Unintentionally, they had shown that analysis of cfDNA could detect an asymptomatic cancer.[5]

At this early stage, cfDNA-based cancer testing has mainly been used for monitoring existing cancer patients for disease recurrence and for guiding the use of drugs that target specific genetic mutations. Over the last few years, though, researchers have been exploring wider applications of these insights to target early detection of cancers.

THE FIRST BLOOD-BASED TESTS REACH THE MARKET

Among the leaders in developing this screening technology are GRAIL and Exact Sciences, although other companies have been developing their own tests and raising significant seed capital to support development of commercial products. Among the companies involved in the field of multicancer blood-based testing are Guardant Health, Freenome, and Delfi Diagnostics.[6]

Exact's test, which the company currently calls its multicancer early-detection test, or MCED, was the first cfDNA early detection assay to be evaluated in a clinical trial. In 2020, before being acquired by Exact, Thrive published results from its DETECT-A study, a 10,000-subject trial.[7] Over the course of two years it identified cancers in twenty-six women. Of those, seventeen had localized cancers that had not spread, and five had stage I disease.

Another study, investigating a prototype of GRAIL's cfDNA pan-cancer test, Galleri, also showed an ability to pick up early-stage tumors, detecting around 17 percent of the stage I cancers in a test group and 40 percent of stage II disease.

What these preliminary tests showed in the studies was that blood-based pan-cancer detection is possible, even if the technologies require further refinement. The developers recommend that the tests be used in addition to the traditional early-detection tests, not in lieu of them. Importantly, these blood-based tests appear to be able to detect tumors for which we currently lack early-detection screening. There is no test, for instance, for three of the stage I cancers discovered in the DETECT-A trial (types of ovarian and uterine tumors). All of these cancers would normally be missed with the current screening technologies, so catching even a small proportion would indicate a serious advance.

Even for lung, breast, and colorectal cancers, for which we already have screening tests, the blood-based tests could ease access and thus increase the rate of use in the general population. And, again, the developers of the tests are recommending that they be used to complement the more traditional, single cancer screening tests.

EASIER ACCESS, LOWER COSTS, GREATER EQUITY

These cfDNA tests offer another potential advantage: simplicity. Any test requires sophisticated chemistry and technologies, but from the patient perspective the blood-based screening is easier to administer than current tests. A simple blood draw is typically all that's required, and that can be done just about anywhere. That is no small thing. Lowering the testing barriers makes it far easier to attract patients and further increases protection for large numbers of people. Lowering testing barriers offers the potential, in theory, of reducing disparities in levels of screening between different population groups. If achieved, that would be particularly meaningful since as the Information Technology and Innovation Foundation report notes, in 2020, African Americans had the highest cancer mortality rates of any racial or ethnic group; cancer is also the leading cause of death among Hispanics, not the generally more prevalent heart disease.[8]

The year after Thrive released its DETECT-A trial data, three GRAIL researchers along with the NCI's Christine Berg (whom we encountered earlier in her role planning for the National Lung Screening Trial, two decades ago) published a study modeling the potential impact of pan-cancer early-detection testing. For the purposes of their analysis, they assumed that the test identified 485 cancers per 100,000 individuals every year. Under that scenario, the incidence of stage III and IV cancers would be reduced by 78 percent and U.S. cancer deaths would be lowered by 26 percent.[9] That is 26 percent of the roughly 600,000 people in the U.S. who die of cancer every year, or more than 150,000 lives saved, an extraordinary outcome.

The performance figures used in this model were based on data from GRAIL's Galleri screening test. In the summer of 2021, the company presented data from another prospective evaluation of the test, called PATHFINDER. The trial involved 6,600 people using the test broken down into two groups—one (comprising 70 percent of the subjects) at high risk of cancer due to factors like genetic predisposition or previous malignancies, and the other (comprising the remaining 30 percent of the group) at average risk.

During the twelve-month study, the Galleri test flagged ninety-two suspected cancers.[10] Of those, thirty-five were determined to be true positives, while fifty-seven were found to be false positives. Of the true positives, nearly half—48 percent—were stage I or II cancers. False positives are, of course, a constant concern with all cancer screening tests and they require careful follow-up.

GRAIL has now put the Galleri test on the market, making it available to patients with a doctor's prescription.

GRAIL is also running an RCT for its Galleri test in collaboration with the U.K.'s National Health Service. It enrolled about 140,000 people between the ages of 50 and 77, half of whom are undergoing testing with Galleri three times over two years. The study won't be looking for cuts in cancer deaths directly, but will try to determine if use of Galleri testing leads to a reduction in the number of late-stage cancers detected. Peter Sasieni, a professor of cancer prevention at King's College London and a leader of the trial, said this would indicate a longer-term mortality benefit to the new screening technology without having to wait many more years to gain data on the actual outcomes.

"We're doing it that way because we want to get results as quickly as possible," Sasieni said. "We believe that if it does lead to a reduction in advanced cancer then we should be thinking about a screening program to [use the test] on a large scale, and we shouldn't wait another two years for mortality data."

In the U.S., the NCI is also planning an RCT that will evaluate several pan-cancer screening tests.

OVERCOMING THE
FALSE POSITIVES CHALLENGE

A key issue for the new blood-based tests, just as it is for the traditional tests, is false positives. Preliminary evidence already indicates
that the pan-cancer tests like Galleri and Exact's MCED perform well
compared to traditional cancer screening tests. For instance, when
administered properly, LDCT lung cancer screening has a false positive rate of about 10 percent. In its trial, Exact's test had a false positive
rate of about 1 percent. Based on the data from the PATHFINDER trial,
the Galleri test also has shown a false positive rate of approximately 1
percent. Those are favorable numbers for widely used screening tests.

The stickier issue is how doctors treat the false positives. In the
case of radiological tests like LCDT lung screening or mammography,
a clinician can see images of any lesions or nodules that are detected. They can then decide to investigate further by employing another
imaging technique or do a biopsy. If they determine that the abnormality does not require urgent treatment, they can wait six months
and then do more imaging to determine if the abnormality has grown
or changed in a dangerous way. The screening allows doctors to focus
their attention with some clarity.

Biochemical tests, such as PSA screening, can be, as we have seen,
more difficult to interpret. An elevated PSA score is just the start of a
process to determine if there is a threat, and how to treat it. Another
test like the 4Kscore can help determine if the initial result was a false
positive or a tumor that can safely go untreated. If there are still questions, an MRI or biopsy may be warranted. If, at the end of it all, the
clinicians do not find any serious abnormalities, they will generally
regard it as a false positive. That does not eliminate the possibility
that, should the elevated PSA level persist, there really is a cancer—
that it is a true positive and the search missed it.

Cell-free-DNA-based cancer testing also faces this challenge.
Consider it from the perspective of a primary care physician. Generally speaking, based on the statistical evidence, for every 1,000 pa-

tients tested doctors will find about ten with positive initial readings, followed by negative results in follow-up screening. For every cancer detected doctors will typically flag between one and five false positives, patients who are subsequently determined to be free of any cancers. Making those determinations accurately and consistently will be key to the effectiveness of any new screening technologies.

There are reasons for optimism, though, based again on the experiences of the trials and the capabilities of the blood-based testing methods. Notably, not only will doctors be able to detect the presence of abnormal DNA in the blood of patients, in the case of the GRAIL test they will be capable of using features of that altered DNA to identify where in the body any tumor is likely to be, with as much as 80 percent accuracy. Furthermore, in the DETECT-A study, doctors found some success in identifying and handling what they determined were false positives.

The first step in the case of a positive blood test was for a panel of experts to review the patient's medical history to consider any potential noncancer causes. If there were none, the patients were given full-body positron emission tomography-computed tomography scans, known as PET scans. That helped confirm the presence of tumors and their location. About 1 percent of participants in the DETECT-A study had PET scan imaging done because of a false positive blood test result. Just 0.22 percent underwent further invasive diagnostic procedures like an endoscopy. Only three patients in the DETECT-A study without cancers underwent surgery, and in all three of those cases doctors found and removed precancerous lesions.

In the PATHFINDER study for GRAIL's Galleri test, seventeen of the fifty-seven patients with false positive cases underwent some sort of invasive procedure as part of the follow-up. In five of these patients, the procedure was administered based on the Galleri test result alone. In the other twelve patients, the decision to administer the invasive procedure was triggered by the positive Galleri result plus either an assessment of the patient's medical history or an additional lab or imaging result. The diagnostic steps and procedures caused no adverse effects.[11]

Jewel Samadder, director of the high-risk cancer clinic at the Mayo Clinic in Arizona, said he has started to see a flow of inquiries from patients either asking him to order the Galleri test or asking him to interpret findings from the test, given increased awareness in response to GRAIL's marketing efforts. But there is still some uncertainty about how exactly to use and interpret the test. Samadder said he has told his Mayo colleagues not to order the test until clearer guidelines around its use are established and implemented. In responding to this new generation of tests, Samadder is leading a Mayo task force doing systematic reviews to determine the appropriate uses.

"We're going to look at all of their published evidence, including meeting abstracts as well as publications, and go through that to create a literature review summary of what data they have in what patient populations, what were the test characteristics in different tumor types, and then work through an algorithm of, if we did, theoretically, use this at Mayo, what patients would we utilize it on, and how would we guide a family practice physician in having a discussion with a patient who comes in saying "I want this test," he said. As of March 2023, Illumina had sold more than 60,000 Galleri tests, generating roughly $55 million of revenue.[12]

NEW TOOLS FOR DETECTING CANCERS MISSED BY OTHER TESTS

The research underway will guide when and how these blood-based tests will be made widely available and, ultimately, how effective they will be. Of the thirty-five cancers detected by Galleri in the PATH-FINDER study, for instance, 71 percent were cancers for which there had previously been no effective screening tests. That is a large multiple of the number of cancer types that can be identified using traditional and well-known early-detection tools alone—mammography, colonoscopy, Pap smear, PSA, LDCT.

When GRAIL looked at results from the first 38,000 Galleri tests it sold commercially, it found the test had flagged 108 individual malignancies spanning twenty-eight cancer types. About 60 percent of those would have gone undetected using the conventional screening methods.[13]

The expectation is that the reliability of the tests will continue to improve as they are refined. Already, the positive initial results are attracting an influx of capital to support the commercial ventures. In addition to GRAIL and Exact, some of the other firms developing pan-cancer screening tests are backed by hundreds of millions of dollars in funding fueled by calculations of the size of the early-detection market. When approved for general use, these early detection tests would have a potentially large global market because of the prevalence of cancer.

Around the world, researchers are hard at work on new technologies for capturing and measuring mutated DNA and other biological markers that signal possible malignances. Some are working on computational techniques to analyze and make sense of this new molecular data.

"There's absolutely lots of runway for improvement," said Kenneth Kinzler, a Johns Hopkins oncologist and one of the founders of Thrive Earlier Detection. Kinzler's research—much of it done with his Johns Hopkins colleague, Bert Vogelstein—has helped lay the foundations for the pan-cancer blood tests.

The science behind many of the new tests is a result of important new insights into how healthy cells work and how cancers hijack or impede those processes. GRAIL's Galleri test works by looking at what is known as DNA methylation. Methylation, a chemical process in which molecular units called methyl groups are attached to DNA, is one way that cells control whether particular genes in the DNA structure are switched on or off, part of a healthy life process.

Cancer occurs when these normal genomic processes are corrupted, distorting their functioning. Abnormal DNA methylation patterns can indicate that a cell's genes are not functioning as they should and that the cell has become malignant. Exact Sciences' MCED test looks at DNA methylation patterns to detect cancer. The test also measures the levels of certain cancer-associated proteins and instances of an abnormality called aneuploidy—a phenomenon common in tumor cells in which the cell either has an extra copy or is missing copies of certain chromosomes.

Other enterprises are researching various approaches to broaden early-detection screening. Delfi Diagnostics, which was founded by another Johns Hopkins oncologist, Victor Velculescu (and includes onetime lung screening skeptic Peter Bach as its chief medical officer), is developing a test for detecting cancer based on unique DNA fragmentation patterns.

Freenome is exploring various cellular features, including DNA methylation, cancer-associated proteins, and RNA, which are the templates cells employ when creating proteins. Recent research suggests that the RNA found in our platelets—cell fragments in blood that stop bleeding—could be employed in other types of pan-cancer screening tests.[14]

THE ECONOMIC STAKES

Cancer, in addition to taking a terrible toll on families and communities, exacts an enormous economic cost on societies, which could be at least partly reversed with reductions in mortality rates. Analysts have estimated the cost of treating cancer comes to 5 percent to 11 percent of the yearly U.S. healthcare budget,[15] and it has been rising sharply, to an estimated $209 billion in 2020, from $190 billion in 2015.[16] Given that cancer is largely a disease of the aged, the federal government, in the form of the Medicare program, covers one-third of the costs.[17]

By removing productive people from the labor force and placing enormous costs on families and the medical system, the burden of cancer on the economy is amplified. A study published in 2008 estimated that, in the year 2000, cancer deaths removed $960.6 billion in economic value.[18]

Those figures underscore why some experts forecast large economic benefits if the medical system can reduce the incidence of the disease and deaths. Kevin Murphy and Robert Topel, in a study in *The Journal of Political Economy*, estimated that even a 1 percent cut in cancer mortality could yield some $500 billion in net present economic benefits.[19] That is another reflection of the benefits of the new early-detection screening technologies if their promise is realized.

Reflecting those prospects, in 2023 a bipartisan group of legislators introduced the Nancy Gardner Sewell Medicare Multi-Cancer Early Detection Screening Coverage Act in the U.S. House of Representatives. The bill, which is named for U.S. Rep. Terri Sewell's mother, who died of pancreatic cancer in 2021, in effect gives the developers of the blood-based screening tests confidence that if they receive FDA approval and bring products to market, Medicare will be able to provide coverage, an essential form of support to assist in rapid adoption.

The bill would also ensure that receiving MCED testing will not impact a person's Medicare coverage for traditional screening tests, allowing MCEDs to complement, as opposed to replace, traditional screening tests. It also provides a similar path to Medicare coverage for future cancer screening tests developed using new or advanced technologies.

The bill's sponsors have argued that passage of the bill would also help reduce disparities in cancer screening between different ethnic, racial, and income groups, lower healthcare costs, and, not least, save significant numbers of lives each year.

If true, all of these steps would signify significant new advances for the necessary revolution in cancer screening.

CHAPTER 11
LAUNCHING THE EARLY-DETECTION REVOLUTION

THE CENTRAL THEME OF THIS BOOK IS THE URGENT NEED TO prioritize early-detection testing as the surest path to radically reducing cancer mortality rates. A comprehensive program that increases the number of at-risk people getting regular cancer screening tests, and thus catching malignancies in their earliest and most treatable stages, would do far more to save and extend lives than all the billions of dollars we currently spend on developing treatments for late-stage disease.

But so far, in our half-century of engagement in the "war on cancer," early detection has been, tragically, a largely missed opportunity, a poor second to the research and spending on those late-stage treatments. Of its $6.4 billion budget for cancer research, treatments, and nonresearch activities, the National Cancer Institute spends a shockingly small 9 percent on detection and diagnostic activities. It is a sadly misguided approach if we are truly determined to turn around our record in stopping cancers and saving lives.

We must face the harsh reality that, despite this massive spending agenda, we have made scant progress in curing or even extending the life of patients with advanced and metastatic cancers. Despite much brilliant science and pioneering medical work, for most of these late-stage cancers, the survival rate hasn't significantly changed over the fifty years since President Nixon launched his anticancer campaign.

Many people mistakenly believe that cancer can often be cured, even at these later stages, and surveys show that high percentages of stage IV cancer patients hold unrealistic expectations of stopping

their disease. While doctors usually want their patients to feel positive and hopeful to assist in their own treatment, these myths can
make it even more challenging to persuade policymakers to allocate a
larger share of NCI and other government health spending to early detection, the best way to achieve significant progress in this great quest.

We are all stakeholders in this debate, all facing the same urgent
need for better answers to problems many of us do not yet know we
have. These are the steps we urge for getting our policy priorities right
and establishing a successful comprehensive strategy for cutting cancer death rates.

1. OUR MOST IMPORTANT PROPOSAL: MORE MONEY

Increasing budgets for solving big policy challenges is at times derided
as ill-conceived or lazy, just "throwing money at the problem," but,
in fueling the early-detection revolution, more funding is essential
and would certainly pay off. Over the years, wisely targeted funding
has provided the foundation for successful screening programs; we
must sharply increase allocations for early-detection campaigns and
research to win the significant benefits they would bring.

Hundreds of thousands could be saved from avoidable early deaths
by increasing the number of people who are regularly screened for
cervical cancer, prostate cancer, breast cancer, colon cancer, and lung
cancer—five common cancers that are responsible for almost half of
cancer deaths and for which we have reliable single-cancer tests. Additional thousands of lives could be saved by developing new screening
tests for other types of cancer, for research that would allow doctors
to distinguish between indolent, nonthreatening malignancies and
aggressive cancers, or by providing better public education to help
patients get proper care after being diagnosed with cancer. All that
requires substantially larger budgets.

Currently, the NCI budget for these measures is woefully inadequate. Dedicating more government investment to these activities would provide an almost immediate payoff. This could be achieved by net increases in budgets, but in this fiscally stressed environment it may be more feasible to reallocate a portion of the NCI and other healthcare budgets to fund major increases in early-detection strategies.

The Centers for Disease Control and Prevention (CDC) is also a central player in this effort. Its mandate includes disease and cancer prevention through its Division of Cancer Prevention and Control, a role that President Joe Biden's Cancer Moonshot initiative has sought to expand. The program, first introduced in 2016, was relaunched in 2022 with a statement from the president that the effort was "a call to action for cancer screening and early detection."[1]

"Today, we know cancer as a disease we often diagnose too late," the Biden administration said in a statement. "We must increase access to existing ways to screen for cancer, and support patients through the process of diagnosis. We can also greatly expand the cancers we can screen for. Five years ago, detecting many cancers at once through blood tests was a dream. Now new technologies and rigorous clinical trials could put this within our reach. Detecting and diagnosing cancers earlier means there may be more effective treatment options."

The White House said, "We can cut the death rate from cancer by at least 50 percent over the next 25 years, and improve the experience of people and their families living with and surviving cancer."

That is laudable, but the time frame—twenty-five years—sets the bar far too low. By contrast, the U.K.'s National Health Service's most recent Long Term Plan committed to increase screening to achieve a goal of detecting 75 percent of the cancer diagnoses in the country at an early stage by 2028.[2] Unquestionably, that would reduce mortality rates significantly, but in one-fifth the time the U.S. promised. It would be a remarkable achievement that the U.S. can and should emulate with aggressive implementation plans and aggressive media campaigns.

Despite the administration's hopeful remarks, the Biden Cancer Moonshot may not provide sufficient funding to fuel significant new progress. The original program provided $1.8 billion over seven years starting in 2017, about an extra $250 million per year, or less than 5 percent of NCI's annual budget.[3] And Congress must now renew that funding to continue the initiative.

In the meantime, funding for major national early-detection programs remains essentially flat. In 2022, Health and Human Services Secretary Xavier Becerra announced $215 million of grants supporting three early-detection programs run by the CDC, but that does not represent a significant increase in support, nor does it promise any game-changing improvements.

For instance, the new funding for one of those programs, the National Breast and Cervical Cancer Early Detection Program, will result in "2,500 additional cancers and cancerous lesions detected," according to the CDC, but that is less than 1 percent of the approximately 300,000 new cases of invasive breast cancer detected each year. That underscores the desperate need for significant increases in funding to reduce mortality rates with truly game-changing initiatives.

Undoubtedly, this rebalancing of the budgets will require a large-scale lobbying effort. But, also undoubtedly, the returns to families, communities, the healthcare system, and the economy would be substantial.

Government will play the largest role in providing the funds necessary for success in the early-detection battle, but the private sector is now contributing growing sums to developing important new early-detection technologies and marketing them.

There has been a surge of private investment in research and development of early-stage cancer diagnostics in recent years. The capital has sparked the formation of numerous start-ups focused on advanced early-detection technologies. The investment is revving up before any new tests have had a significant impact on the early-detection struggle. The excitement is about potential.

Take the example of Exact Sciences, which produces the colorectal cancer screening test Cologuard as well as the multicancer early-detection test originally developed by Thrive Earlier Detection. In 2020, Exact spent more than $550 million on research and development of early-detection technologies[4] and another $400 million in 2021.[5] That's comparable to what the NCI spends annually supporting early-detection research.

It still is not up to the vast spending levels of the Big Pharma companies—for instance, Merck spends around $2 billion a year on R&D,[6] though only a portion of that goes to oncology—but it is rising to levels that make breakthroughs and better uptake more likely.

2. USE EVERY ARROW IN THE MEDIA AND MARKETING QUIVER

Of the five widely employed early-detection tests, lung cancer screening is the least used. This is puzzling and highly regrettable, since lung cancer kills 130,000 people a year, one-quarter of all cancer deaths. Yet only 4.5 percent of those at greatest risk—smokers and former smokers in their 50s and older—get screened.

We have highlighted the reasons behind the failure to employ the early-detection test for lung cancer, LDCT, more widely, despite clear evidence that it saves lives. The National Committee for Quality Assurance (NCQA), the organization that sets the influential healthcare provider performance standards, Healthcare Effectiveness Data and Information Set, or HEDIS, has not yet included lung cancer screening as an essential element of a good healthcare plan, which means there is less incentive for healthcare providers to offer this critical service. If the NCQA were to include LDCT in HEDIS, adoption of this critical test would likely increase and the efforts to reduce cancer mortality rates would receive a big boost.

But there is a way to provide an even larger boost. Well-funded information and publicity campaigns, including use of current social media, advertising, and marketing programs, have proven over and over that they can raise awareness of the benefits of screening and improve uptake. The best example is the CDC's Screen for Life initiative, which has sharply increased use of colorectal cancer screening over the past twenty years.

This initiative has included numerous focus groups to fine-tune the messaging, the use of $300 millions' worth of public service ads to spread the word, and the employment of celebrities like Katie Couric to endorse this important early-detection test. Over the roughly two decades during which the campaign has run, the percentage of U.S. residents up to date with recommended colorectal cancer screenings has nearly doubled, to more than two-thirds of the population, from about one-third. It provides a model that should be emulated for other early-detection tests, especially for lung cancer.

We know these smart targeted campaigns work for another reason: the big pharmaceutical companies rely heavily on such marketing and spend billions of dollars a year on them because they are so effective.

3. ELIMINATE DISPARITIES IN SCREENING AND TREATMENT RATES

Cancer affects all kinds of people, in all age, income, ethnic, and racial groups, but its burdens fall disproportionately on disadvantaged groups—lower-income people, Blacks and Hispanics, rural residents. The disparities are well documented. These issues of race, language, income, health insurance coverage, education, and employment mean those underserved communities suffer lower screening rates and, generally, higher mortality rates from cancer. Once cancer has been detected, patients from these groups often run into delays in treatment or get less-effective treatments, if they get specialized care at all.

These differences are unjust and unacceptable, and we have allowed them to persist too long. They represent a weak front in the war on cancer. But the problems can be remedied.

The use of patient navigators has proven an effective means of reducing some of these disparities. However, the lack of meaningful insurance reimbursement for patient navigator services reduces the number of guides that have been deployed. This coverage gap can and should be fixed with regulations and, if needed, legislation. Importantly, efforts must be made to get Medicare and Medicaid to support patient navigators, which, in the long term, save the healthcare system money. And HEDIS must include the use of patient navigators as one metric in determining the ranking of health plans.

Another model for reducing disparities was developed during the AIDS crisis. In 1990, Congress passed the Ryan White Comprehensive AIDS Resources Emergency (CARE) Act, which, among other measures, expanded care for lower-income and uninsured people with HIV/AIDS, providing primary medical care and other support services for uninsured or underinsured individuals living with HIV. The program has proven very successful, and it could serve as a model for reducing disparities in cancer screening and treatment for disadvantaged groups.

The Ryan White Act focuses not only on medical treatment but also provides funding to cities, states, and other entities to support services like nutrition care, mental health services, transportation, and case management. The act also funds programs aimed at education and awareness about HIV/AIDS. Similarly, programs that increase education and awareness about the importance of early cancer detection should be funded and expanded, targeting underserved communities.

4. BETTER TRAINING OF CARE PROVIDERS AND TECHNICIANS

In early detection, rigorous and regular training for providers and deep experience matter a great deal. Many providers, whether primary care physicians or specialists, are still skeptical of early detection, at times due to outdated information or a poor understanding of the protocols for assessing results and following up. Better training and improved information campaigns would, as a first step, help providers understand the processes needed for using the tests properly to identify malignancies and treat them. Doctors need to understand the highly complex issues involved in interpreting test results and the procedures that should be followed to address inevitable complications such as false positives and false negatives. Experience drives the process.

A study done by Peter Scardino, a urologist, surgeon, and expert on prostate cancer at the Memorial Sloan-Kettering Cancer Center, found that prostate cancer patients treated by inexperienced surgeons had a nearly 70 percent higher risk of recurrence within five years than patients treated by highly experienced surgeons.[7] And doctors must be highly proficient in cancer screening literacy so they can explain to patients the benefits and potential problems with screening. This requires a deep familiarity with the science behind the screening protocols and the statistical evidence on screening.

Another area of importance in screening is imaging. Screening often depends on imaging, including mammograms, LDCT tests, MRIs, PET scans, and ultrasounds. Lawrence Schwartz, chair of radiology at Memorial Sloan-Kettering, notes that it can be difficult to read these images and ascertain imaging errors, because there are many different types, and they can be directed at many different parts of the body. As a result, error rates can vary widely, from just a few percent to multiples of that.

To combat these challenges, some European countries require providers to read a minimum number of images a year for certification at levels much higher than in the U.S. The U.S., for instance, requires only that providers do 480 readings a year to be qualified to read mammograms, compared with 5,000 annually in the U.K.[8] Additionally, in much of Europe it is common for labs and hospitals to require a second reader of imaging like mammograms. The U.S. needs to raise its standards for certification to improve quality and reliability.

5. FUND RESEARCH INTO THE NEW GENERATION OF EARLY-DETECTION TESTS

The most important pioneering work being done for early detection is in multicancer screening. These tests hold the promise of simplifying screening, allowing providers to test for numerous cancer types with one draw of blood, and of detecting early-stage cancers for which we currently have no tests. If they succeed, they would be immensely important breakthrough technologies with the potential for transforming the cancer battle. Private investors are pouring money into some of the companies working on these protocols, but the government should also make this research a high priority. It is hard to imagine any area providing a better return on investment than these new pan-cancer technologies.

Researchers need to focus on increasing the accuracy and sensitivity of the tests—reducing both false negatives and false positives—while successful implementation will require making sure that providers and technicians are well trained in how to decipher results and properly follow them up, and take steps to make sure that, when fully developed, the costs of the tests are covered by Medicare, Medicaid, and commercial insurers.

Our understanding of cancer as well as the cellular mechanisms that cancer corrupts has vaulted ahead in recent decades. But few of those discoveries have been more important in helping us defeat the disease than learning how to detect abnormalities early before they grow and spread. We will, if we succeed in expanding adoption of precise and reliable new early-detection tests, save millions more lives. That is what makes early detection such a high priority and promising public health objective.

None of this is easy. We have outlined many of the financial, medical, human, and procedural challenges that the expansion of early detection faces. But one thing the history of early detection and the research supports is optimism. Addressing disparities and guaranteeing access to screening can significantly enhance the effectiveness of early-detection protocols, ensuring that all people, no matter their background, benefit from these advances. A comprehensive approach that prioritizes patient needs, enhances medical literacy, funds cutting-edge research, and encourages strategic collaborations will produce the radically lower mortality rates that have, so far in the war on cancer, eluded us.

They are now within reach.

ACKNOWLEDGEMENTS

FROM MY EARLIEST DAYS AS A YOUNG PUBLIC INTEREST LAWYER *and then as New York City's Commissioner of Consumer Affairs under Mayor Ed Koch, I've been passionate about using the best research and data as the foundation for effective public policy. Even as I later pursued a career in property development, I continued this cause by joining the boards of the Memorial Sloan-Kettering Cancer Center and Weill Cornell Medicine, two institutions that epitomize the philosophy of applying innovative science to saving lives and improving public health. These positions, which I have now held for several decades, have been enormously rewarding because of the remarkable work by the leadership and professionals at the institutions. They inspired me to work hard to understand their research and their successes, and I want to thank them for their generous efforts to assist me in understanding their work on cancer care. Those relationships have made my life immensely richer.*

Through this work I came to appreciate that, despite the brilliant work being done in trying to defeat cancer, our policies are out of balance and not reducing death rates nearly as much as they should. That is how I concluded that the best way finally to start winning our war against this terrible disease is by placing much greater emphasis on early detection screening, the theme of this book. All the proceeds from this book are being donated to cancer-focused nonprofit organizations.

One of the most inspirational physician-scientists I have known and perhaps the greatest influence on my understanding of the importance of early detection has been Peter Scardino. Peter was chairman of both the Department of Urology at Memorial Sloan-Kettering and its Department of Surgery. He is a brilliant surgeon and clinician and drilled into me the importance of early detection of cancer based on his philosophy of putting patients' interests first.

I also owe a debt of gratitude to another physician-scientist who inspired me to write this book, José Baselga. During a conversation in April 2016, José, who was physician-in-chief and chief medical officer at Memorial Sloan-Kettering, told me about new research that had demonstrated that it might be possible to detect cancer at a very early stage through a blood test for what is known as cell-free DNA. DNA from tumor cells, he explained, is shed into the bloodstream and can be identified through gene sequencing.

His description of this eye-opening new technology was the initial impetus for me to learn more about how we might save lives by catching cancer early. José died at 61 in 2021, a great loss to his field. He was a visionary in working to make cancer a controllable chronic condition rather than a deadly disease.

Philip Stieg, a highly respected professor and chairman of Weill Cornell Medical College's Department of Neurological Surgery, was a pioneer in thinking about and developing tests for the early detection of brain tumors, other abnormalities, and dangerous medical conditions. He has been a friend and adviser on how we can take imaging directly into communities through mobile scanners. Lisa DeAngelis, the chief physician executive at Memorial Sloan-Kettering, has given me a much better understanding of cancer and cancer research during the many years that I have served on the board. Her judgment and interest in patient care have been models for me and helped me appreciate the importance of always considering and placing the highest priority on the patient's well-being.

Two other physician-scientists, Claudia Henschke and David Yankelewitz at Mt. Sinai Hospital in New York, have probably saved more lives of lung cancer victims than any other scientist or doctor through their efforts to expand adoption of LDCT screening. I am grateful for the advice and help that Claudia and David have given me in learning about LDCT technology.

When I decided to run a pilot program with a mobile lung cancer screening device in 2019, I reached out to Robert Min, chairman of the Department of Radiology at Weill Cornell Medicine, and Bradley Pua, division chief of Interventional Radiology. We successfully ran a four-week program giving free LDCT scans in downtown Brooklyn. This helped us develop a better understanding of how to expand adoption of this important technology.

José Guillem, formerly a gastrointestinal surgeon at Memorial Sloan-Kettering and now chief of the Division of Gastrointestinal Surgery at the University of North Carolina School of Medicine, encouraged me to write this book and was always available for advice as well as reading drafts.

Lawrence Schwartz, chair of the Department of Radiology at Memorial Sloan-Kettering, helped me understand the issues around imaging and early detection, including suggestions on how to reduce reader errors as well as ways to increase the use of LDCT scans.

Luiz Diaz Jr., the head of the Division of Solid Tumor Oncology at Memorial Sloan-Kettering and a creative scientist, strongly believes in the need for expanding early detection efforts. We consulted him as we began this book and have continued to discuss ideas on how we can detect more cancers in their earliest stages.

Two friends have also been invaluable. Dick Beattie, senior chairman of the law firm Simpson Thacher & Bartlett and former chairman of the board of Memorial Sloan-Kettering, has devoted much of his life to civic duty, supporting numerous meaningful organizations that have improved the lives of untold numbers of the less advantaged. He is a close and kind friend who has read drafts of the book, made many helpful suggestions, and, importantly, recommended to us our editor and collaborator, James Sterngold. Jim spent many years as an award-winning reporter and foreign correspondent with The New York Times *and* The Wall Street Journal *and has done an excellent job sharpening the book. He made many valuable suggestions on content, organization, and style. I am grateful for his wisdom and guidance.*

Glenn Dopf, probably the best medical malpractice defense attorney in New York City, read the original outline and drafts of the book and provided many helpful comments. He also introduced me to many physicians and scientists.

I also offer my thanks and respect to my co-author, Adam Bonislawski. Adam is a science writer with more than ten years' experience covering genomic and proteomic research and diagnostics development with the online publications GenomeWeb and 360DX. I have been working with Adam on this project for five years and he has done an excellent job as a researcher and interviewer.

My gratitude also goes to my publisher, Colin Robinson, CEO and co-founder of OR Books. I appreciate that Colin embraced a first-time author and provided so much help in getting the book into print.

I am fortunate to have a wonderful family that has supported this project from the start. My wife, Linda Johnson, who is the CEO of the Brooklyn Public Library and a leader in assisting underserved communities, has been an encouraging champion of this book. Her matchless reading and writing skills and her willingness to take the time to critique this book has improved it greatly. My daughter, Rebbie Ratner, has always been supportive and has taken a keen interest in early detection of cancer and was the perfect person to discuss many of the issues in this book. My daughter Lizzy Ratner, deputy editor at The Nation *magazine, has helped us organize the book and worked with Jim Sterngold on the editing. She is a superb journalist and editor.*

As a property developer, I had the honor of working with and getting to know the architect Frank Gehry, who designed for us a skyscraper in downtown Manhattan. He was kind enough to design the cover of this book.

My daily working partner and collaborator is Aryeh Baraban, a mathematician who has worked as a schoolteacher and a business risk manager. Aryeh introduced me to Adam, runs my office, directed our pilot project on mobile screening for lung cancer, and contributed to my thinking about early detection. Cynthia McCollum, the senior vice president of hospital administration at Memorial Sloan-Kettering, discussed with us many times both how to increase screening and reduce the disparities in cancer care.

This has been a team effort. I could not have undertaken this project without the generous support of the many talented doctors and scientists who kindly provided their time and insights to finally win the war on cancer.

—Bruce Ratner

EARLY DETECTION IS AN ENORMOUSLY COMPLICATED FIELD,
which means this book has necessarily relied on the advice and expertise of
many talented, brilliant, and, above all, busy people. I'm indebted to them for
their time and patience in answering my many questions and helping me to
better understand the field.

I won't tax the reader's patience with the full list of the researchers and
physicians, administrators, and policymakers who took the time to speak with
me for the book. But the contributions of a few must be singled out. Claudia
Henschke and David Yankelevitz took me through the intricacies of lung can-
cer screening and the clinical trial process. Andrea and Brady McKee and
their Lahey Clinic colleagues detailed their work pioneering an LDCT pro-
gram. Harold Freeman recounted his role as the developer of patient naviga-
tion; Andrew Vickers and Peter Scardino helped me understand the ins and
outs of PSA and prostate cancer screening; and Stephen Grubbs told me the
story of Delaware's Screening for Life program.

Maria Fernandez and her work helped me better understand how access
is just one of many challenges to implementing cancer screening, while Shelley
Hwang, Victoria Seewaldt, and Elizabeth Morris showed me the seemingly end-
less complexities of mammography and breast cancer screening. Steven Woolf
was an invaluable resource on the early days of the USPSTF as well as many
other points on early detection. I thank them and all the many, many others
without whose help the book would not have been possible.

Finally, thanks to my wife, Rachel Feierman, for her support, encourage-
ment, and love throughout.

—Adam Bonislawski

NOTES

INTRODUCTION

1. American Cancer Society, "Cancer Facts & Figures 2022." https://www
.cancer.org/content/dam/cancer-org/research/cancer-facts-and-statistics/
annual-cancer-facts-and-figures/2022/2022-cancer-facts-and-figures.pdf.

2. C.C. Boring, T.S. Squires, and T. Tong, "Cancer Statistics, 1991," *Boletín de
la Asociación Médica de Puerto Rico* 83, no. 6 (June 1991): 225–42.

3. American Cancer Society, "Survival Rates for Colorectal Cancer," accessed
2022; revised March 1, 2023, https://www.cancer.org/cancer/colon-rec-
tal-cancer/detection-diagnosis-staging/survival-rates.html.

4. American Cancer Society, "Survival Rates for Breast Cancer," accessed
2022; revised March 1, 2023, https://www.cancer.org/cancer/breast-cancer/
understanding-a-breast-cancer-diagnosis/breast-cancer-survival-rates.html.

5. American Cancer Society, "Survival Rates for Prostate Cancer," accessed
2022; revised March 1, 2023, https://www.cancer.org/cancer/prostate-can-
cer/detection-diagnosis-staging/survival-rates.html.

6. "Can We Prevent Cancer? Yes, Says Bert Vogelstein, If We Try Harder,"
YouTube, uploaded by Breakthrough, August 22, 2016, //www.youtube.com/
watch?v=RoYkCnbFBrQ.

7. "Nixing Colon Cancer: The Hilton-Ludwig Cancer Prevention Initiative,"
Ludwig Link (September 2015): 3, //www.ludwigcancerresearch.org/
wp-content/uploads/2020/10/LudwigLink_September-2015.pdf.

CHAPTER 1

1. Cristian Tomasetti and Bert Vogelstein, "Variation in Cancer Risk Among
Tissues Can Be Explained by the Number of Stem Cell Divisions," *Science*
347, no. 6217 (January 2, 2015): 78–81.

2. "Can We Prevent Cancer? Yes, Says Bert Vogelstein, If We Try Harder," YouTube, uploaded by Breakthrough, August 22, 2016, //www.youtube.com/watch?v=RoYkCnbFBrQ.

3. ESMO, "ESMO-Magnitude of Clinical Benefit Scale Scorecards" (January 2020), //www.esmo.org/guidelines/esmo-mcbs/esmo-mcbs-scorecards.

4. R.S Herbst, P. Baas, D.W. Kim, et al., "Pembrolizumab versus docetaxel for previously treated, PD-L1-positive, advanced non-small-cell lung cancer (KEYNOTE-010): a randomised controlled trial," *Lancet* 387, no. 10027 (April 9, 2016): 1540–50, https://doi.org/10.1016/S0140-6736(15)01281-7.

5. J.C. Weeks, P.J. Catalano, A. Cronin, M.D. Finkelman, J.W. Mack, N.L. Keating, and D. Schrag, "Patients' Expectations about Effects of Chemotherapy for Advanced Cancer," *New England Journal of Medicine* 367, no. 17 (October 25, 2012): 1616–25, //doi.org/10.1056/NEJMoa1204410.

6. A. Cercek, M. Lumish, J. Sinopoli, et al., "PD-1 Blockade in Mismatch Repair-Deficient, Locally Advanced Rectal Cancer," *New England Journal of Medicine* 386, no. 25 (June 23, 2022): 2363–76, //doi.org/10.1056/NEJMoa2201445.

7. Gina Kolata, "A Cancer Trial's Unexpected Result: Remission in Every Patient." *New York Times,* June 5, 2022, //www.nytimes.com/2022/06/05/health/rectal-cancer-checkpoint-inhibitor.html.

8. National Cancer Institute, "Funding Allocated to Major NCI Program Areas," Posted May 10, 2022, //www.cancer.gov/about-nci/budget/factbook/data/program-structure.

9. Centers for Disease Control and Prevention, "FY 2021 Operating Plan," PDF dated February 19, 2021, //www.cdc.gov/budget/documents/fy2021/FY-2021-CDC-Operating-Plan.pdf.

10. American Cancer Society, "American Cancer Society 2020 Annual Report," undated PDF, //www.cancer.org/content/dam/cancer-org/online-documents/en/pdf/reports/2020-annual-report.pdf.

11. *Conquest of Cancer Act: Hearings,* before the Senate Comm. on Labor and Public Welfare, Subcomm. on Health, 92nd Cong., 200 (1971).

12. *Conquest of Cancer Act:* Hearings, 219 (1971).

13. *Conquest of Cancer Act:* Hearings, 219 (1971).

14. American Lung Association, *"State of Lung Cancer 2023 – Lung Cancer Key Findings,"* https://www.lung.org/research/state-of-lung-cancer/key-findings.

15. Z. Berkowitz, X. Zhang, T.B. Richards, M. Nadel, L.A. Peipins, and J. Holt, "Multilevel Small-Area Estimation of Colorectal Cancer Screening in the United States," *Cancer Epidemiol Biomarkers & Prevention 27,* no. 3 (March 2018): 245–253, //doi.org/10.1158/1055-9965.EPI-17-0488.

16. Z. Berkowitz, X. Zhang, T.B. Richards, S.A. Sabatino, L.A. Peipins, J. Holt, and M.C. White, "Multilevel Regression for Small-Area Estimation of Mammography Use in the United States, 2014," *Cancer Epidemiol Biomarkers & Prevention 28*, no. 1 (January 2019): 32–40, //doi.org/10.1158/1055-9965. EPI-18-0367.

17. S.H. Woolf and R.E. Johnson, "The Break-Even Point: When Medical Advances Are Less Important than Improving the Fidelity with Which They Are Delivered," *Annals of Family Medicine 3*, no. 6 (November 2005): 545–52, //doi.org/10.1370/afm.406.

18. R.C. Brownson, P. Allen, R.R. Jacob, J.K. Harris, K. Duggan, P.R. Hipp, and P.C. Erwin, "Understanding Mis-Implementation in Public Health Practice," *American Journal of Preventive Medicine* 48, no. 5 (May 2015): 543–51, //doi .org/10.1016/j.amepre.2014.11.015.

CHAPTER 2

1. D. Erskine Carmichael, *The Pap Smear—Life of George N. Papanicolaou* (Springfield, Illinois: Charles C. Thomas, 1973), vii.

2. Romanian physician Aurel Babes discovered around the same time that he could detect the presence of cervical cancer by examining cells collected using a platinum loop, but history has generally credited Papanicolaou with inventing the procedure.

3. Carmichael, *The Pap Smear,* 44–5.

4. Carmichael, *The Pap Smear,* 59–60.

5. Heinz Grunze and Arthur Spriggs, eds., *History of Clinical Cytology* (Darmstadt, Germany: GIT Verlag Ernst Giebler, 1980), 90.

6. Grunze and Spriggs, *Clinical Cytology,* 80.

7. Carmichael, *The Pap Smear,* 68–9.

8. Carmichael, *The Pap Smear,* 71.

9. Carmichael, *The Pap Smear,* 75–6.

10. Carmichael, *The Pap Smear,* 76.

11. Carmichael, *The Pap Smear,* 76.

12. U.S. Congress House Comm. on Appropriations, 85th Congress, Vol. 16, 412 (1958).

13. 1978 NCI Fact Book, National Cancer Institute, U.S. Department of Health, Education, and Welfare (December 1978), NIH Publication No. 79–512, 40.

14. M.J. Casper and A.E. Clarke, "Making the Pap Smear into the 'Right Tool' for the Job," *Social Studies of Science* 28, no. 3 (April 1998): 255–90, //doi.org/10.1177/030631298028002003.

15. Laura Pelehach, "Appraising the Pap Smear," *Laboratory Medicine* 28, no. 7 (1997): 440.

16. Speaking of Women's Health, "Cervical Cancer Screening Guidelines," https://speakingofwomenshealth.com/health-library/cervical-cancer-screening-guidelines.

17. Laura Pelehach, "The Pap Smear on Trial," Laboratory Medicine 28, no. 8 (1997): 511.

18. Casper and Clarke, "Making the Pap Smear," 255–90.

19. *Clinical Laboratories: Hearings before the Subcomm. on Oversight and Investigations of the House Comm. on Energy and Commerce,* 100th Cong. (1988), (testimony of Shirley Greening, professor of cytotechnology and cytogenetics at Thomas Jefferson University in Philadelphia).

20. *Clinical Laboratories: Hearings before the Subcomm. on Oversight and Investigations of the House Comm. on Energy and Commerce,* 100th Cong. (1988), (testimony of the American Society for Cytotechnology).

21. G.S. Ogilvie, D. van Niekerk, M. Krajden, et al., "Effect of Screening with Primary Cervical HPV Testing vs Cytology Testing on High-grade Cervical Intraepithelial Neoplasia at 48 Months: The HPV FOCAL Randomized Clinical Trial," *JAMA* 320, no. 1 (July 3, 2018): 43–52, //doi.org/10.1001/jama.2018.7464.

22. H.G. Rosenblum, R.M. Lewis, J.W. Gargano, T.D. Querec, E.R. Unger, and L.E. Markowitz, "Declines in Prevalence of Human Papillomavirus Vaccine-Type Infection Among Females after Introduction of Vaccine—United States, 2003–2018." *Morbidity and Mortality Weekly Report* 70, no. 12 (March 26, 2021): 415–20, //www.cdc.gov/mmwr/volumes/70/wr/mm7012a2.htm.

CHAPTER 3

1. C.I. Henschke, D.I. McCauley, D.F. Yankelevitz, D.P. Naidich, G. McGuinness, O.S. Miettinen, D.M. Libby, et al., "Early Lung Cancer Action Project: overall design and findings from baseline screening," *Lancet* 354, no. 9173 (July 10, 1999): 99–105, //doi.org/10.1016/S0140-6736(99)06093-6.

2. Denise Grady, "CAT Scan Process Could Cut Deaths From Lung Cancer." *New York Times,* July 9, 1999, //www.nytimes.com/1999/07/09/us/cat -scan-process-could-cut-deaths-from-lung-cancer.html. Accessed September 26, 2019.

3. Henschke, et al., "Early Lung Cancer Action Project."

4. A.A. Vaporciyan, M.S. Kies, C.W. Stevens, et al., "Factors Associated with the Development of Lung Cancer," in *Holland-Frei Cancer Medicine,* 6th edition, ed. D.W. Kufe, R.E. Pollock, R.R. Weichselbaum, et al., (Hamilton, Ontario: B.C. Decker, 2003), chap. 92.

5. National Cancer Institute, "Cancer Stat Facts: Lung Cancer," //seer.cancer .gov/statfacts/html/lungb.html.

6. National Cancer Institute, "Cancer Stat Facts," //seer.cancer.gov/ statfacts/html/lungb.html.

7. G.Z. Brett, "The Value of Lung Cancer Detection by Six-Monthly Chest Radiographs," *Thorax* 23, no. 4 (July 1968): 414–20, //doi.org/10.1136/ thx.23.4.414.

8. M.R. Melamed, B.J. Flehinger, M.B. Zaman, R.T. Heelan, W.A. Perchick, and N. Martini, "Screening for Early Lung Cancer. Results of the Memorial Sloan-Kettering Study in New York," *Chest* 86, no. 1 (July 1984): 44–53, //doi.org/10.1378/chest.86.1.44.

9. M. Tockman, "Survival and Mortality from Lung Cancer In a Screened Pop-ulation," *Chest* 89, no. 4 (April 1986): 324S–325S, //journal.chestnet.org/ article/S0012-3692(16)61988-8/fulltext.

10. R.S. Fontana, D.R. Sanderson, L.B. Woolner, W.F. Taylor, W.E. Miller, and J.R. Muhm, "Lung Cancer Screening: The Mayo Program," *Journal of Occupational Medicine 28,* no. 8 (August 1986): 746–50, //doi .org/10.1097/00043764-198608000-00038.

11. A. Kubík and J. Polák, "Lung Cancer Detection. Results of a Randomized Prospective study in Czechoslovakia," *Cancer* 57, no. 12 (June 15, 1986): 2427–37, //doi.org/10.1002/1097-0142(19860615)57: 12<2427: : aid -cncr2820571230>3.0.co;2-m.

12. M.M. Oken, W.G. Hocking, P.A. Kvale, G.L. Andriole, S.S. Buys, T.R. Church, E.D. Crawford, et al., "Screening by Chest Radiograph and Lung Cancer Mortality: The Prostate, Lung, Colorectal, and Ovarian (PLCO) Randomized Trial," *JAMA* 306, no. 17 (November 2, 2011): 1865–73, //doi.org/10.1001/ jama.2011.1591.

13. L.R. Goodman, "The Beatles, the Nobel Prize, and CT Scanning of the Chest," *Radiologic Clinics of North America* 48, no. 1 (January 2010): 1–7, //doi.org/10.1016/j.rcl.2009.09.008.

14. M. Kaneko, K. Eguchi, H. Ohmatsu, R. Kakinuma, T. Naruke, K. Suemasu, and N. Moriyama, "Peripheral Lung Cancer: Screening and Detection with low-Dose Spiral CT Versus Radiography," *Radiology* 201, no. 3 (December 1996): 798–802, //doi.org/10.1148/radiology.201.3.8939234.

15. S. Sone, S. Takashima, F. Li, Z. Yang, T. Honda, Y. Maruyama, M. Hasegawa, T. Yamanda, K. Kubo, K. Hanamura, and K. Asakura, "Mass Screening for Lung Cancer with Mobile Spiral Computed Tomography Scanner," *Lancet* 351, no. 9111 (April 25, 1998): 1242–5, //doi.org/10.1016/S0140-6736(97)08229-9.

16. P.B. Bach, "Response to 'CT Screening for Lung Cancer: Update 2007,'" *The Oncologist* 13, no. 5 (May 2008): 608–09, https://doi.org/10.1634/the-oncologist.2008-0031.

17. O.S. Miettinen, "Screening for Lung Cancer: Do We Need Randomized Trials?" *Cancer* 89, no. 11, supplement (December 7, 2000): 2449–52, //doi.org/10.1002/1097-0142(20001201)89: 11+<2449: : AID-CNCR20>3.0.CO;2-8.

18. National Lung Screening Trial Research Team, D.R. Aberle, A.M. Adams, C.D. Berg, W.C. Black, J.D. Clapp, R.M. Fagerstrom, et al., "Reduced Lung-Cancer Mortality with low-Dose Computed Tomographic Screening," *New England Journal of Medicine* 365, no. 5 (August 4, 2011): 395–409, //doi.org/10.1056/NEJMoa1102873.

19. Medicare Evidence Development & Coverage Advisory Comm. (April 30, 2014), (testimony of Paul Pinksy).

20. P.B. Bach, "Inconsistencies in Findings from the Early Lung Cancer Action Project Studies of Lung Cancer Screening," *Journal of the National Cancer Institute* 103, no. 13 (June 17, 2011): 1002–6, //doi.org/10.1093/jnci/djr202.

21. Bach, Peter, "CT Scam," *Slate*, Nov. 15, 2010, //slate.com/technology/2010/11/not-everyone-should-get-screened-for-lung-cancer-using-ct-scans.html, accessed October 5, 2019.

22. Denise Grady, "A.I. Took a Test to Detect Lung Cancer. It Got an A," *New York Times,* May 20, 2019, //www.nytimes.com/2019/05/20/health/cancer-artificial-intelligence-ct-scans.html.

23. Eric Topol, Twitter, May 20, 2019, //twitter.com/erictopol/status/1130495794451116032.

24. Otis Brawley, "CMS Got it Right," The Cancer Letter 40, no. 43 (November 14, 2014): 1,5, //cancerletter.com/paid/20141114_2/.

25. American Lung Association, "What to Expect from a Lung Cancer Screening." //www.lung.org/lung-health-diseases/lung-disease-lookup/lung-cancer/saved-by-the-scan/resources/what-to-expect-from-lung-cancer-screening.

26. D. Sackett, "A 1955 Clinical Trial Report that Changed My Career," *Journal of the Royal Society of Medicine* 103, no. 6 (2010): 254–5, //doi.org/10.1258/jrsm.2010.10k003.

27. G.H. Guyatt, "Evidence-based medicine," ACP *Journal Club* (March/April 1991): A-16, //doi.org/10.7326/ACPJC-1991-114-2-A16.

28. *Medicare Evidence Development & Coverage Advisory Comm.* (April 30, 2014), (testimony of Peter Bach).

29. *Medicare Evidence Development & Coverage Advisory Comm.* (April 30, 2014), (testimony of Steven Woolf).

30. H.J. de Koning, C.M. van der Aalst, P.A. de Jong, E.T. Scholten, K. Nackaerts, M.A. Heuvelmans, J.J. Lammers, et al., "Reduced Lung-Cancer Mortality with Volume CT Screening in a Randomized Trial," *New England Journal of Medicine* 382, no. 6 (February 6, 2020): 503–13, //doi.org/10.1056/NEJMoa1911793.

31. Henschke CI, Yip R, Shaham D, et al., "A 20-year Follow-up of the International Early Lung Cancer Action Program (I-ELCAP)," *Radiology* 309, no. 2 (November 7, 2023): e231988. //doi:10.1148/radiol.231988.

32. U.S. Preventive Services Task Force, A.H. Krist, K.W. Davidson, C.M. Mangione, M.J. Barry, M. Cabana, A.B. Caughey, et al., "Screening for Lung Cancer: US Preventive Services Task Force Recommendation Statement," *JAMA* 325, no. 10 (March 9, 2021): 962–70, //doi.org/10.1001/jama.2021.1117.

33. Chan Yeu Pu, Christine M. Lusk, Christine Neslund-Dudas, et al., "Comparison Between the 2021 USPSTF Lung Cancer Screening Criteria and Other Lung Cancer Screening Criteria for Racial Disparity in Eligibility," *JAMA Oncology* 8, no. 3 (2022): 374–382, //doi.org/10.1001/jamaoncol.2021.6720.

34. D.E. Wood, E.A. Kazerooni, S.L. Baum, et al., "Lung Cancer Screening, Version 3.2018, Clinical Practice Guidelines in Oncology," *Journal of National Comprehensive Cancer Network* 16, no. 4 (2018): 412–41, //doi.org/10.6004/jnccn.2018.0020.

35. David S. Gierada, William C. Black, Caroline Chiles, Paul F. Pinsky, and David F. Yankelevitz, "Low-Dose CT Screening for Lung Cancer: Evidence from 2 Decades of Study," *Radiology: Imaging Cancer 2*, no. 2 (March 27, 2020), //doi.org/10.1148/rycan.2020190058.

CHAPTER 4

1. A.R. Rao, H.G. Motiwala, and O.M. Karim, "The Discovery of Prostate-Specific Antigen," *BJU International* 101, no. 1 (August 30, 2007): 5–10, //doi.org/10.1111/j.1464-410X.2007.07138.x.

2. T.A. Stamey, N. Yang, A.R. Hay, J.E. McNeal, F.S. Freiha, and E. Redwine, "Prostate-Specific Antigen as a Serum Marker for Adenocarcinoma of the Prostate," *New England Journal of Medicine* 317, no. 15 (October 8, 1987): 909–16, //doi.org/10.1056/NEJM198710083171501.

3. J.L. Jahn, E.L. Giovannucci, and M.J. Stampfer, "The High Prevalence of Undiagnosed Prostate Cancer at Autopsy: Implications for Epidemiology and Treatment of Prostate Cancer in the Prostate-Specific Antigen-era," *International Journal of Cancer* 137, no. 12 (December 29, 2014): 2795–2802, //doi.org/10.1002/ijc.29408.

4. Richard Ablin, *The Great Prostate Hoax* (New York, New York: St. Martin's Press, 2014), 43.

5. Weill Cornell Medicine, "Incidence of Metastatic Prostate Cancer in Older Men Increases Following Drop in PSA Screening," news release, December 29, 2016, //news.weill.cornell.edu/news/2016/12/incidence-of-metastatic-prostate-cancer-in-older-men-increases-following-drop-in-psa.

6. U.S. Preventive Services Task Force, "Screening for Prostate Cancer: U.S. Preventive Services Task Force Recommendation Statement," *Annals of Internal Medicine* 149, no. 3 (August 5,2008): 185–91, //doi.org/10.7326/0003-4819-149-3-200808050-00008.

7. F.H. Schröder, J. Hugosson, M.J. Roobol, et al., "Screening and Prostate Cancer Mortality: Results of the European Randomised Study of Screening for Prostate Cancer (ERSPC) at 13 years of follow-up," *Lancet* 384, no. 9959 (August 6, 2014): 2027–35, //doi.org/10.1016/S0140-6736(14)60525-0.

8. P.F. Pinsky, P.C. Prorok, K. Yu, B.S. Kramer, A. Black, J.K. Gohagan, E.D. Crawford, et al., "Extended Mortality Results for Prostate Cancer Screening in the PLCO Trial with Median Follow-up of 15 Years," *Cancer* 123, no. 4 (December 1, 2016): 592–99, //doi.org/10.1002/cncr.30474.

9. A. Tsodikov, R. Gulati, E.A.M. Heijnsdijk, P.F. Pinsky, S.M. Moss, S. Qiu, T.M. de Carvalho, et al., "Reconciling the Effects of Screening on Prostate Cancer Mortality in the ERSPC and PLCO Trials," *Annals of Internal Medicine* 167, no. 7 (October 3, 2017): 449–55, //doi.org/10.7326/M16-2586.

10. B.A. Mahal, S. Butler, I. Franco, D.E. Spratt, T.R. Rebbeck, A.V. D'Amico, and P.L. Nguyen, "Use of Active Surveillance or Watchful Waiting for Low-Risk Prostate Cancer and Management Trends Across Risk Groups in the United States, 2010-2015,) *JAMA* 321, no. 7 (February 11, 2019): 704–6, //doi.org/10.1001/jama.2018.19941.

11. American Cancer Society, "Survival Rates for Prostate Cancer," (accessed March 1, 2022; updated March 1, 2023), //www.cancer.org/cancer/prostate-cancer/detection-diagnosis-staging/survival-rates.html.

12. A. Vickers, S. Carlsson, V. Laudone, and H. Lilja, "It Ain't What You Do, It's the Way You Do It: Five Golden Rules for Transforming Prostate-Specific Antigen Screening," *European Urology* 66, no. 2 (August 2014): 188–90, //doi.org/10.1016/j.eururo.2013.12.049.

13. A.J. Vickers, F.J. Bianco, A.M. Serio, J.A. Eastham, D. Schrag, E.A. Klein, A.M. Reuther, et al., "The Surgical Learning Curve for Prostate Cancer Control after Radical Prostatectomy," *Journal of the National Cancer Institute* 99, no. 15 (August 1, 2007): 1171–7, //doi.org/10.1093/jnci/djm060.

14. C.J. Savage and A.J. Vickers, "Low Annual Caseloads of United States Surgeons Conducting Radical Prostatectomy," *Journal of Urology* 182, no. 6 (December 2009): 2677–79, //doi.org/10.1016/j.juro.2009.08.034.

15. D.J. Parekh, S. Punnen, D.D. Sjoberg, S.W. Asroff, J.L. Bailen, J.S. Cochran, R. Concepcion, et. al., "A Multi-Institutional Prospective Trial in the USA Confirms that the 4Kscore Accurately Identifies Men with High-Grade Prostate Cancer, *European Urology* 68, no. 3 (September 2015): 464–70,. //doi.org/10.1016/j.eururo.2014.10.021.

16. I.G. Schoots, "MRI in Early Prostate Cancer Detection: How to Manage Indeterminate or Equivocal PI-RADS 3 Lesions?" *Translational Andrology and Urology* 7, no. 1 (February 23, 2018): 70¬–82, //doi.org/10.21037/tau.2017.12.31.

17. A.N. Giaquinto, H. Sung, K.D. Miller, J.L. Kramer, L.A. Newman, A. Minihan, A. Jemal, and R.L. Siegel, "Breast Cancer Statistics, 2022," CA: *A Cancer Journal for Clinicians* 72, no. 6 (October 3, 2002): 524–41, //doi.org/10.3322/caac.21754.

18. J. Yu, R.H. Nagler, E.F. Fowler, K. Kerlikowske, and S.E. Gollust, "Women's Awareness and Perceived Importance of the Harms and Benefits of Mammography Screening: Results From a 2016 National Survey," *JAMA Internal Medicine* 177, no. 9 (September 2017): 1381–2, https://doi.org/10.1001/jamainternmed.2017.2247.

19. J. Gershon-Cohen, M.B. Hermel, and S.M. Berger, "Detection of Breast Cancer by Periodic X-Ray Examinations. A Five-Year Survey," *JAMA* 176, no. 13 (July 1, 1961): 1114–6, https://doi.org/10.1001/jama.1961.63040260015013a.

20. S. Shapiro, P. Strax, and L. Venet, "Periodic Breast Cancer Screening in Reducing Mortality From Breast Cancer," *JAMA* 215, no. 11 (March 15, 1971): 1777–85, https://doi.org/10.1001/jama.1971.03180240027005.

21. Handel Reynolds, *The Big Squeeze* (Ithaca, New York: Cornell University Press, 2012).

22. L. Esserman, Y. Shieh, and I. Thompson, "Rethinking Screening for Breast Cancer and Prostate Cancer," *JAMA* 302, no. 15 (October 21, 2009): 1685–92, https://doi.org/10.1001/jama.2009.1498.

23. A. Bleyer and H.G. Welch, "Effect of Three Decades of Screening Mammography on Breast-Cancer Incidence," *New England Journal of Medicine* 367, no. 21 (November 22, 2012): 1998–2005, https://doi.org/10.1056/NEJMoa1206809.

24. A.L. Siu, U.S. Preventive Services Task Force, "Screening for Breast Cancer: U.S. Preventive Services Task Force Recommendation Statement," *Annals of Internal Medicine* 164, no. 4 (February 16, 2016): 279–96, https://doi.org/10.7326/M15-2886.

25. J.G. Elmore, M.B. Barton, V.M. Moceri, S. Polk, P.J. Arena, and S.W. Fletcher, "Ten-Year Risk of False Positive Screening Mammograms and Clinical Breast Examinations," *New England Journal of Medicine* 338, no. 16 (April 16, 1998): 1089–96, https://doi.org/10.1056/NEJM199804163381601.

26. A.L. Siu, U.S. Preventive Services Task Force, "Screening for Breast Cancer," 279–96, https://doi.org/10.7326/M15-2886.

27. U.S. Preventive Services Task Force, "Breast Cancer: Screening" (May 2023), https://www.uspreventiveservicestaskforce.org/uspstf/draft-recommendation/breast-cancer-screening-adults.

28. R.M. Mann, A. Athanasiou, P.A.T. Baltzer, et al., "Breast Cancer Screening in Women with Extremely Dense Breasts Recommendations of the European Society of Breast Imaging (EUSOBI)," *European Radiology* 32 (March 8, 2022): 4036–45, //doi.org/10.1007/s00330-022-08617-6.

29. Centers for Disease Control and Prevention, "What Does It Mean to Have Dense Breasts?" (September 26, 2022), https://www.cdc.gov/cancer/breast/basic_info/dense-breasts.htm.

30. S.H. Busch, J.R. Hoag, J.A. Aminawung, et al., "Association of State Dense Breast Notification Laws With Supplemental Testing and Cancer Detection After Screening Mammography," *American Journal of Public Health* 109, no. 5 (May 2019): 762–67, https://doi.org/10.2105/AJPH.2019.304967.

31. J. Melnikow, J.J. Fenton, E.P. Whitlock, et al., "Supplemental Screening for Breast Cancer in Women With Dense Breasts: A Systematic Review for the U.S. Preventive Service Task Force [Internet]. Rockville (MD): Agency for Healthcare Research and Quality (US); 2016 Jan. (Evidence Syntheses, No. 126.)

32. L. Salvatorelli, L. Puzzo, G.M. Vecchio, R. Caltabiano, V. Virzì, and G. Magro, "Ductal Carcinoma In Situ of the Breast: An Update with Emphasis on Radiological and Morphological Features as Predictive Prognostic Factors, *Cancers* (Basel) 12, no. 3 (March 6, 2020): 609, https://doi.org/10.3390/cancers12030609.

33. M. van Seijen, E.H. Lips, A.M. Thompson, S. Nik-Zaina, A. Futreal, E.S. Hwang, E. Verschuur, et al., "Ductal Carcinoma in Situ: To Treat or Not to Treat, that Is the Question," *British Journal of Cancer* 121, no. 4 (July 9, 2019): 285–92, https://doi.org/10.1038/s41416-019-0478-6.

34. K. Kerlikowske, "Epidemiology of Ductal Carcinoma in Situ," *Journal of the National Cancer Institute Monographs* 2010, no. 41 (October 2010): 139–41, https://doi.org/10.1093/jncimonographs/lgq027.

35. F.C. Hamdy, J.L. Donovan, J.A. Lane, M. Mason, C. Metcalfe, P. Holding, M. Davis, T.J. Peters, et al., "10-Year Outcomes after Monitoring, Surgery, or Radiotherapy for Localized Prostate Cancer," *New England Journal of Medicine* 375, no. 15 (October 13, 2016): 1415–24. //doi.org/10.1056/ NEJMoa1606220.

36. S. Hofvind, S. Thoresen, and S. Tretli, "The Cumulative Risk of a False-Positive Recall in the Norwegian Breast Cancer Screening Program," *Cancer* 101, no. 7 (September 14, 2004): 1501–7, //doi.org/10.1002/ cncr.20528.

37. X. Castells, E. Molins, and F. Macià, "Cumulative False Positive Recall Rate and Association with Participant Related Factors In A Population Based Breast Cancer Screening Programme," *Journal of Epidemiology and Community Health* 60, no. 4 (2006): 316–21, //doi.org/10.1136/jech.2005.042119.

38. C.D. Lehman, R.F. Arao, B.L. Sprague, J.M. Lee, D.S. Buist, K. Kerlikowske, L.M. Henderson, et al., "National Performance Benchmarks for Modern Screening Digital Mammography: Update from the Breast Cancer Surveillance Consortium," *Radiology* 283, no. 1 (April 2017): 49–58, //doi .org/10.1148/radiol.2016161174.

39. U.S. Food and Drug Administration, "MQSA National Statistics," March 3, 2022; page updated May 1, 2023, //www.fda.gov/radiation-emitting-products/mqsa-insights/mqsa-national-statistics.

40. A. Chong, S.P. Weinstein, E.S. McDonald, and E.F. Conant, "Digital Breast Tomosynthesis: Concepts and Clinical Practice," *Radiology* 292, no. 1 (May 14, 2019): 1–14, //doi.org/10.1148/radiol.2019180760.

41. D.S.M. Buist, L. Abraham, C.I. Lee, J.M. Lee, C. Lehman, E.S. O'Meara, N.K. Stout, et al., "Breast Biopsy Intensity and Findings Following Breast Cancer Screening in Women With and Without a Personal History of Breast Cancer," *JAMA Internal Medicine* 178, no. 4 (April 2018): 458–468, //https://doi.org/10.1001/jamainternmed.2017.8549.

42. C. Printz, "Most Women Have an Inaccurate Perception of Their Breast Cancer Risk," Cancer 120, no. 3 (January 22, 2014): 314–5, //doi .org/10.1002/cncr.28557.

CHAPTER 5

1. NORC at the University of Chicago, "Only 14% of Cancers Are Detected Through a Preventive Screening Test," December 14, 2022, https://www.norc.org/ content/dam/norc-org/pdfs/State-Specific%20PCDSs%20chart%201213.pdf.

2. I. Lansdorp-Vogelaar, K.M. Kuntz, A.B. Knudsen, M. van Ballegooijen, A.G. Zauber, A. Jemal, "Contribution of Screening and Survival Differences to Racial Disparities in Colorectal Cancer Rates," *Cancer Epidemiol Biomarkers and Prevention* 21, no. 5 (2012): 728–36, https://doi.org/10.1158/1055 -9965.EPI-12-0023.

3. M.E. Fernández, L.S. Savas, K.M. Wilson, T.L. Byrd, J. Atkinson, I. Tor-res-Vigil, and S.W. Vernon, "Colorectal Cancer Screening among Latinos in Three Communities on the Texas-Mexico Border," *Health Education & Behavior* 42, no. 1 (February 2015): 16–25, https://doi .org/10.1177/1090198114529592.

4. E.M. Roncancio, K.K. Ward, I.A. Sanchez, M.A. Cano, T.L. Byrd, S.W. Ver-non, M.E. Fernandez-Esquer, et al., "Using the Theory of Planned Behavior to Understand Cervical Cancer Screening Among Latinas," *Health Education & Behavior* 42, no. 5. (October 2015): 621–6. https://doi .org/10.1177/1090198115571364.

5. "Addressing the Screening Gap: The National Breast and Cervical Cancer Early Detection Program: Hearing Before the Comm. on Oversight and Gov-ernment Reform," House of Representatives, 110th Cong., Second Session, January 29, 2008 (United States: U.S. Government Printing Office): 88.

6. G. Neta, M.A. Sanchez, D.A. Chambers, et al., "Implementation Science in Cancer Prevention and Control: A Decade of Grant Funding by the National Cancer Institute and Future Directions," *Implementation Science* 10, article 4 (January 8, 2015), https://doi.org/10.1186/s13012-014-0200-2.

7. National Cancer Institute, "Implementation Science Centers in Cancer Control (ISC3)," June 17, 2021, https://cancercontrol.cancer.gov/is/ initiatives/isc3.

8. A. DeGroff, A. Carter, K. Kenney, Z. Myles, S. Melillo, J. Royalty, K. Rice et al., "Using Evidence-Based Interventions to Improve Cancer Screening in the National Breast and Cervical Cancer Early Detection Program," *Journal of Public Health Management & Practice* 22, no. 5 (September–October 2016): 442–9, https://doi.org/10.1097/PHH.0000000000000369.

9. K. Kenney, A. Carter, S. Melillo, and A. Satsangi, "Evaluating Changes in the Use of Evidence-Based Interventions in the National Breast and Cervical Cancer Early Detection Program" (presented at the Prevent Cancer Founda-tion Dialogue for Action Conference, Baltimore, MD, April 6–8, 2016).

10. R.C. Brownson, P. Allen, R.R. Jacob, J.K. Harris, K. Duggan, P.R. Hipp, and P.C. Erwin PC. "Understanding Mis-Implementation in Public Health Prac-tice," *American Journal of Preventive Medicine* 48, no. 5 (May 2015): 543–51, https://doi.org/10.1016/j.amepre.2014.11.015.

11. National Cancer Institute, "Colorectal Cancer Screening," April 2022, https://progressreport.cancer.gov/detection/colorectal_cancer.

12. National Cancer Institute, "Cancer Stat Facts: Colorectal Cancer," https://seer.cancer.gov/statfacts/html/colorect.html.

13. Centers for Disease Control and Prevention, "Screen for Life: National Colorectal Cancer Action Campaign," February 3, 2022, https://www.cdc .gov/cancer/colorectal/sfl/about.htm.

14. C. Beeker, J.M. Kraft, B.G. Southwell, and C.M. Jorgensen, "Colorectal Cancer Screening in Older Men and Women: Qualitative Research Findings and Implications for Intervention," *Journal of Community Health* 25, no. 3 (June 2000): 263–78, https://doi.org/10.1023/a: 1005104406934.

15. C.M. Jorgensen, C.A. Gelb, T.L. Merritt, and L.C. Seeff, "Observations from the CDC: CDC's Screen for Life: A National Colorectal Cancer Action Campaign," *Journal of Women's Health & Gender-Based Medicine* 10, no. 5 (June 2001): 417–22, https://doi.org/10.1089/152460901300233876.

16. C.P. Cooper, C.A. Gelb, H. Jameson, E. Macario, C.M. Jorgensen, and L. Seeff, "Developing English and Spanish Television Public Service Announcements to Promote Colorectal Cancer Screening, *Health Promotion Practice* 6, no. 4 (October 2005): 385–93, https://doi .org/10.1177/1524839905278759.

17. Beth Snyder Bulik, "The Top 10 Ad Spenders in Big Pharma for 2020," *Fierce Pharma,* April 2021, https://www.fiercepharma.com/special-report/ top-10-ad-spenders-big-pharma-for-2020.

18. Bulik, "Top 10 Ad Spenders," https://www.fiercepharma.com/special -report/top-10-ad-spenders-big-pharma-for-2020.

19. Bristol Myers Squibb, *2020 Annual Report,* March 2020, https://s27 .q4cdn.com/119407475/files/doc_downloads/2021/BMY_2020Financial-Report.pdf.

CHAPTER 6

1. S.F. Oluwole, A.O. Ali, A. Adu, B.P. Blane, B. Barlow, R. Oropeza, and H.P. Freeman, "Impact of a Cancer Screening Program on Breast Cancer Stage at Diagnosis in a Medically Underserved Urban Community," *Journal of the American College of Surgeons* 196, no. 2 (February 2003): 180–8. https:// doi.org/10.1016/S1072-7515(02)01765-9.

2. "A summary of the American Cancer Society Report to the Nation: Cancer in the Poor," CA: A Cancer Journal for Clinicians 39, no. 5 (September–October 1989): 263–5, https://doi.org/10.3322/canjclin.39.5.263.

3. U.K. Henschke, L.D. Leffall Jr., C.H. Mason, A.W Reinhold, R.L. Schneider, and J.E. White, "Alarming Increase of the Cancer Mortality in the U.S. Black Population (1950–1967)," *Cancer* 31, no. 4 (April 1973): 763–8, https://doi.org/10.1002/1097-0142(197304)31:4<763::AID-CN -CR2820310401>3.0.CO;2-S.

4. K. Rice, L. Gressard, A. DeGroff, J. Gersten, J. Robie, S. Leadbetter, R. Glover-Kudon, and L. Butterly, "Increasing Colonoscopy Screening in Disparate Populations: Results from an Evaluation of Patient Navigation in the New Hampshire Colorectal Cancer Screening Program," *Cancer* 123, no. 17 (September 1, 2017): 3356–66, https://doi.org/10.1002/cncr.30761.

5. K. Hede, "Agencies Look to Patient Navigators to Reduce Cancer Care Disparities," Journal of the National Cancer Institute 98, no. 3 (February 1, 2006): 157–9, https://doi.org/10.1093/jnci/djj059.

6. K. Rice, K. Sharma, C. Li, L. Butterly, J. Gersten, and A. DeGroff, "Cost-Effectiveness of a Patient Navigation Intervention to Increase Colonoscopy Screening among Low-Income Adults in New Hampshire," *Cancer* 125, no. 4 (February 15, 2019): 601–9, https://doi.org/10.1002/cncr.31864.

7. David Balderson and Kaveh Safav, "How Patient Navigation Can Cut Costs and Save Lives," *Harvard Business Review,* March 19, 2013, https://hbr. org/2013/03/how-patient-navigation-brings.

8. https://www.congress.gov/bill/117th-congress/housebill/9285?s=1&r=1.

9. Margie Patlak, Cyndi Trang, and Sharyl J. Nass, *Establishing Effective Patient Navigation Programs in Oncology: Proceedings of a Workshop* (Washington, D.C.: The National Academies Press, 2018), 72–73.

CHAPTER 7

1. T.A. Battaglia, K.M. Freund, J.S. Haas, N. Casanova, S. Bak, H. Cabral, R.A. Freedman, K.B. White, et al., "Translating Research into Practice: Protocol for a community-Engaged, Stepped Wedge Randomized Trial to Reduce Disparities in Breast Cancer Treatment through a Regional Patient Navigation Collaborative," *Contemporary Clinical Trials* 93 (June 2020): 106007, https://doi.org/10.1016/j.cct.2020.106007.

2. "Development of Patient Navigation Programs and Their Role in Promoting Health Literacy—Session 5: Mandi Pratt-Chapman," Video, YouTube, uploaded by NASEM Health and Medicine Division, July 30, 2019, https://www.youtube.com/watch?v=C8-iajxDnpl.

3. Elizabeth H. Bradley and Lauren A. Taylor, *The American Health Care Paradox: Why Spending More is Getting Us Less* (New York: PublicAffairs, 2013).

4. A.H. Krist, K.W. Davidson, Q. Ngo-Metzger, J. Mills, "Social Determinants as a Preventive Service: U.S. Preventive Services Task Force Methods," *American Journal of Preventive Medicine* 57, no. 6 (December 2019): S6–S12, https://doi.org/10.1016/j.amepre.2019.07.013.

5. L.M. Nichols and L.A. Taylor, "Social Determinants as Public Goods: A New Approach to Financing Key Investments in Healthy Communities," *Health Affairs* 37, no. 8 (August 2018): 1223–1230, https://doi.org/10.1377/hlthaff.2018.0039.

CHAPTER 9

1. NCQA, "NCQA Health Insurance Plan Ratings 2019–2020—Summary Report (Private/Commercial)," https://healthinsuranceratings.ncqa.org/2019/Default.aspx.

2. J.R. Moehr, "To Morris F. Collen: Happy Ninetieth!" *Journal of the American Medical Informatics Association* 10, no. 6 (November 2003): 613–15, https://doi.org/10.1197/jamia.m1438.

3. J.V. Selby, G.D. Friedman, C.P. Quesenberry Jr., and N.S. Weiss, "A Case-Control Study of Screening Sigmoidoscopy and Mortality from Colorectal Cancer," *New England Journal of Medicine* 326, no. 10 (March 5, 1992): 653–57, https://doi.org/10.1056/NEJM199203053261001.

4. Rickey Hendricks, *A Model For National Health Care: The History of Kaiser Permanente* (New Brunswick, New Jersey: Rutgers University Press, 1993), 26–27.

5. K.F. Rhoads, M.I. Patel, Y. Ma, and L.A. Schmidt, "How do integrated Health Care Systems Address Racial and Ethnic Disparities in Colon Cancer?" *Journal of Clinical Oncology* 33, no. 8 (March 10, 2015): 854–860, https://doi.org/10.1200/JCO.2014.56.8642.

6. M.H. Kanter, J.E. Schottinger, and R. Copeland, "Integration Alone Does Not Reduce Health Care Disparities," *Journal of Clinical Oncology* 33, no. 30 (October 20, 2015): 3519, https://doi.org/10.1200/JCO.2015.61.5047.

7. J. Crosson, "Dr Garfield's Enduring Legacy—Challenges and Opportunities," *Permanente Journal* 10, no. 2 (June 1, 2006): 40–45. https://doi.org/10.7812/tpp/05-146.

8. National Cancer Institute, "State Cancer Profiles." https://statecancerprofiles.cancer.gov/index.html.

9. Surveillance, Epidemiology, and End Results (SEER) Program (www.seer.cancer.gov), SEER*Explorer database, "Colon and Rectum Recent Trends in U.S. Age-Adjusted Mortality Rates, 2000–2019," U.S. Mortality Files, National Center for Health Statistics, CDC.

10. S.S. Grubbs, B.N. Polite, J. Carney Jr., et al., "Eliminating Racial Disparities in Colorectal Cancer in the Real World: It Took a Village," *Journal of Clinical Oncology* 31, no. 16 (June 1 2013): 1928–30, https://doi.org/10.1200/JCO.2012.47.8412.

11. Delaware Health and Social Services, Division of Public Health, "Behavioral Risk Factor Survey (BRFS)," 2018.

12. National Center for Health Statistics, CDC, "Cancer Mortality by State, 2020," (February 28, 2022), https://www.cdc.gov/nchs/pressroom/sosmap/cancer_mortality/cancer.htm.

13. National Cancer Institute, "State Cancer Profiles," https://statecancerprofiles.cancer.gov/index.html.

14. Delaware Health & Social Services, Division of Public Health, "Cancer Incidence And Mortality In Delaware" 2015–2019, https://www.dhss.delaware.gov/dhss/dph/dpc/files/im2015_2019.pdf.

CHAPTER 10

1. Remarks of Bert Vogelstein, "The Multi-Cancer Early Detection Screening Coverage Act Webinar," March 10, 2021.

2. Stephen Ezell, "Seizing the Transformative Opportunity of Multi-Cancer Early Detection," Information Technology and Innovation Foundation, April 2021, https://itif.org/publications/2021/04/19/seizing-transformative-opportunity-multi-cancer-early-detection/.

3. Cancer Research UK, "Why Is Early Cancer Diagnosis Important?" https://www.cancerresearchuk.org/about-cancer/spot-cancer-early/why-is-early-diagnosis-important.

4. Christina A. Clarke, "Projected Reductions in Absolute Cancer-Related Deaths from Diagnosing Cancers Before Metastasis, 2006–2015," *Cancer Epidemiology, Biomarkers, and Prevention* 29, no. 5 (May 2020): 895–902, https://cebp.aacrjournals.org/content/29/5/895.

5. C.M. Osborne, E. Hardisty, P. Devers, K. Kaiser-Rogers, M.A. Hayden, W. Goodnight, and N.L. Vora, "Discordant Noninvasive Prenatal Testing Results in a Patient Subsequently Diagnosed with Metastatic Disease," *Prenatal Diagnosis* 33, no. 6 (June 2013): 609–11, https://doi.org/10.1002/pd.4100.

6. Ezell, "Seizing the Transformative Opportunity," https://itif.org/publications/2021/04/19/seizing-transformative-opportunity-multi-cancer-early-detection/.

7. A.M. Lennon, A.H. Buchanan, I. Kinde, et al., "Feasibility of Blood Testing Combined with PET-CT to Screen for Cancer and Guide Intervention," *Science* 369, no. 6499 (April 28, 2020): eabb9601, https://doi.org/10.1126/science.abb9601.

8. The National Minority Quality Forum, "National Minority Quality Forum Urges Action in Multi-Cancer Early Detection," news release, December 4, 2020, https://https://www.nmqf.org/nmqf-media/mced.

9. E. Hubbell, C.A. Clarke, A. Aravanis, and C.D. Berg, "Modeled Reductions in Late-Stage Cancer with a Multi-Cancer Early Detection Test," *Cancer Epidemiology, Biomarkers & Prevention* 30, no. 3 (March 2021): 460–468, https://doi.org/10.1158/1055-9965.EPI-20-1134.

10. D. Schrag, C.H. McDonnell III, L. Nadauld, C.A. Dilaveri, E.A. Klein, R. Reid, C.R. Marinac, et. al., "A Prospective Study of a Multi-Cancer Early Detection Blood Test," *Annals of Oncology* 33, suppl. 7 (2022): S417–S426, https://doi.org/10.1016/j.annonc.2022.07.1029.

11. GRAIL, "GRAIL Announces Final Results From the PATHFINDER Multi-Cancer Early Detection Screening Study at ESMO Congress 2022," news release, September 11, 2022, https://grail.com/press-releases/grail-announces-final-results-from-the-pathfinder-multi-cancer-early-detection-screening-study-at-esmo-congress-2022/.

12. Illumina, "Illumina Underscores Commitment to Shareholder Value and Responds to Carl Icahn's Statements," news release, March 20, 2023, https://www.illumina.com/company/news-center/press-releases/2023/dd63723d-f082-450c-957d-3192988c76d3.html.

13. GRAIL, "GRAIL Announces Final Results," https://grail.com/press-releases/grail-announces-final-results-from-the-pathfinder-multi-cancer-early-detection-screening-study-at-esmo-congress-2022/.

14. S.G.J.G. In 't Veld, M. Arkani, E. Post, et al., "Detection and Localization of Early- and Late-Stage Cancers Using Platelet RNA," *Cancer Cell* 40, no. 9 (September 1, 2022): 999–1009.e6, https://doi.org/10.1016/j.ccell.2022.08.006.

15. Matthew P. Banegas, et al., "Medical Care Costs Associated With Cancer in Integrated Delivery Systems," *Journal of the National Comprehensive Care Network* 16, no. 4 (April 2018): 402–9, https://doi.org/10.6004/jnccn.2017.7065.

16. National Cancer Institute, "Financial Burden of Cancer Care," April 2022, https://progressreport.cancer.gov/after/economic_burden.

17. Andrew Shooshtari, Yamini Kalidindi, and Jeah Jung, "Cancer Care Spending and Use by Site of Provider-Administered Chemotherapy in Medicare," *American Journal of Managed Care* 25, no. 6 (June 14, 2019), https://www.ajmc.com/view/cancer-care-spending-and-use-by-site-of-provideradministered-chemotherapy-in-medicare.

18. K. Robin Yabroff, "Estimates and Projections of Value of Life Lost From Cancer Deaths in the United States," *Journal of the National Cancer Institute* 100, no. 24 (December 17, 2008): 1755–62, https://doi.org/10.1093/jnci/djn383.

19. Kevin Murphy and Robert Topel, "The Value of Health and Longevity," Journal of Political Economy 114, no. 5 (October 2006): 871–904, https://doi.org/10.1086/508033.

CHAPTER 11

1. Joseph Biden, "Remarks by President Biden at an Event to Reignite the Cancer Moonshot," The White House, Washington, D.C., February 2, 2022, https://www.whitehouse.gov/briefing-room/speeches-remarks/2022/02/02/remarks-by-president-biden-at-an-event-to-reignite-the-cancer-moonshot/.

2. NHS England, "NHS Long Term Plan," January 2019, https://www.longtermplan.nhs.uk/publication/nhs-long-term-plan/. Page updated August 2019.

3. Joseph Biden, "Remarks by President Biden at an Event to Reignite the Cancer Moonshot," February 2, 2022.

4. Exact Sciences, Form 10-K annual report filing for 2020 with the Securities and Exchange Commission, February 16, 2021, https://d18rn0p25nwr6d.cloudfront.net/CIK-0001124140/b80b06a8-ab85-4451-a931-0f350e003edd.pdf.

5. Exact Sciences, Form 10-K annual report filing for 2021 with the Securities and Exchange Commission, February 22, 2022, https://d18rn0p25nwr6d.cloudfront.net/CIK-0001124140/36d3687b-6084-4031-9b54-9f609c-bc6e32.pdf.

6. Merck, 2020 *Annual Report,* March 2021, https://www.emdgroup.com/en/annualreport/2020/.

7. A.J. Vickers, F.J. Bianco, A.M. Serio, J.A. Eastham, D. Schrag, E.A. Klein, A.M. Reuther, et al., "The Surgical Learning Curve for Prostate Cancer Control after Radical Prostatectomy," *Journal of the National Cancer Institute* 99, no. 15 (August 1, 2007): 1171–7, https://doi.org/10.1093/jnci/djm060.

8. NHS England, "Breast Screening: Guidance for Image Reading," February 16, 2023, https://www.gov.uk/government/publications/breast-screening-guidance-for-image-reading/breast-screening-guidance-for-image-reading.

INDEX